# Chesneys' Equipment for Student Radiographers

# Chesneys' Equipment for Student Radiographers

Fourth Edition

**Peter Carter**

with

**Audrey Paterson**

**Mike Thornton**

**Andrew Hyatt**

**Andrew Milne**

**John Pirrie**

**Blackwell**
Science

Editorial Offices:
Blackwell Science Ltd, 9600 Garsington Road, Oxford OX4 2DQ, UK
Tel: +44 (0) 1865 776868
Blackwell Publishing Inc., 350 Main Street, Malden, MA 02148-5020, USA
Tel: +1 781 388 8250
Blackwell Science Asia Pty, 550 Swanston Street, Carlton, Victoria 3053, Australia
Tel: +61 (0)3 8359 1011

First edition published 1971
Second edition published 1975
Third edition published 1984
Fourth edition published 1994

8    2006

ISBN-13: 978-0-632-02724-8
ISBN-10: 0-632-02724-X

Library of Congress Cataloging-in-Publication Data
Chesneys' equipment for student radiographers/P.H. Carter ... [et al.].—4th ed.
    p.    cm.
    Rev. ed. of: X-ray equipment for student radiographers/D. Noreen Chesney. 1984.
    Includes bibliographical references and index.
    ISBN  0-632-02724-X
    1. Radiography, Medical—Equipment and supplies.    I. Carter, P.H. (Peter H.)    II.
Chesney, D. Noreen. X-ray equipment for student radiographers.
    RC78.5.C48    1994
    616.07'572—dc20
93-40039
CIP

A catalogue record for this title is available from the British Library

The publisher's policy is to use permanent paper from mills that operate a sustainable forestry policy, and which has been manufactured from pulp processed using acid-free and elementary chlorine-free practices. Furthermore, the publisher ensures that the text paper and cover board used have met acceptable environmental accreditation standards.

For further information on
Blackwell Publishing, visit our website:
www.blackwellpublishing.com

# Contents

# List of Contributors

**Peter Carter**, *BEd (Hons)*, *MA*, *FCR*, *TDCR*, *Cert Ed*. Principal Lecturer, Sheffield Hallam University.

**Andrew Hyatt**, *BA*, *DNM*, *TDCR*, Senior Lecturer, Sheffield Hallam University.

**Andrew Milne**, *DMS*, *DCR*, Superintendent Radiographer, Northern General Hospital, Sheffield.

**Audrey Paterson**, *MSc*, *TDCR*, *DMU*, Head of Department of Radiography, Canterbury Christ Church College.

**John Pirrie**, *DMS*, *TDCR*, Senior Lecturer, Sheffield Hallam University.

**Mike Thornton**, *BA*, *TDCR*, Senior Lecturer, Leeds College of Health.

# Preface to the First Edition

This is not the book we planned to write. When we began it the idea was to produce a book about diagnostic X-ray equipment which would be simple, primarily concerned with practicalities and reassuringly short. Instead we have a book which – we believe – should be reasonably easy to understand; we are encouraged in this respect by a physicist friend who is half-inclined to think it is too simple. It *is* very much concerned with the actual use of X-ray equipment. It is not, however, short.

Modern diagnostic apparatus is not a small subject, and perhaps we were foolish to believe that a brief manual on it could be written at a level likely to be useful to those who are presently preparing for the diploma examinations of the Society of Radiographers and always required to put to good use the expensive toys in their departments. We have tried to make every word in this book count, and we hope that student readers will not be intimidated by its appearance of length.

So far as we know this is the first book to be written about the subject called Diagnostic X-ray Equipment in the Society of Radiographers' syllabus for its qualifying diploma. True, X-ray equipment is included in other works but it is mixed with physics or radiographic technique. Because we enjoy using and understanding – if we can – properly designed apparatus, and because too few radiographers teach this subject in their schools, we have believed there is a place for a book that will concentrate on what X-ray equipment does, and provide basic explanations that may be helpful not only to students but perhaps also to the radiographers who teach them. We recognize that some of the topics in this book have been adequately covered elsewhere, for example the X-ray tube, but we would submit also that others have not appeared before in a formal textbook for radiographers, at least in the English language.

Because we wished to make the book one from which it is easy to learn, we have tried to avoid complexity in its many diagrams, especially in the circuit diagrams. This means that in various instances the drawings do not represent complete working arrangements and we make no apology for this, since their aim is to provide understanding and not to facilitate an X-ray installation.

Some references to physics have been essential, but we have generally assumed in our readers a certain knowledge of these matters and have limited our own probings as much as we can. Such subjects as electronoptics have been treated in relation to their application to a specific piece of equipment rather than in an academic context. This we believe to be the right approach because we are sure that the study of diagnostic X-ray equipment – if it is to be useful to radiographers – should be practical, its place the X-ray room as much as the classroom.

While the Society of Radiographers' syllabus for its qualifying diploma has established guidelines for the writing of this book, there are nevertheless matters here which do not appear in the present syllabus, though they are much in evidence in X-ray departments. It is therefore necessary to teach them to students and for post-diploma radiographers to have some understanding of them. We hope that both these groups of people will be helped by our small forays into television, electronics and other present advances in radiological equipment.

Perhaps the best part of writing the preface to a textbook is being able to say 'Thank you' to those from whom we have freely drawn assistance. That we have confidence in this book is due to the help of our friends among physicists and manufacturers of X-ray equipment who not only have given us much of their expensive time and unfailingly answered all our questions, but have not seemed to mind doing so. Our expert team of readers were Mr R.F. Farr, Chief Physicist at the United Birmingham Hospitals; Mr C.W. Mead of Watson and Sons (Electro-Medical) Ltd (GEC Medical Equipment Ltd); Mr J.E. Steadman, who was then working with A.E. Dean and Co. (GEC Medical Equipment Ltd); Mr G. Waters of Machlett X-ray Tubes (Great Britain) Ltd (GEC Medical Equipment Ltd). Mr C.J. Hills, also of Watson and Sons, was let off lightly and kindly read Chapter 9. We hope that he did not regard his subsequent departure from the United Kingdom as an escape. Chapter 11 profited from the advice of Mr L.A. Newman of Philips Electrical Ltd. We are immeasurably grateful to them all. Their knowledge has provided this book with its sinews and their kindness has given to the writing of it a special reward.

We are grateful for the use of illustrative material supplied to us by several organizations. In particular we appreciate the energy displayed in our cause by Mr David Scott when he was Publicity Manager of Watson & Sons (Electro-Medical) Ltd, and by Mr Malcolm Holmes, Publicity Manager of GEC Medical Equipment Ltd. The following have permitted us to publish photographs and diagrams belonging to them and it is a pleasure here to record our appreciation of this assistance: Barr and Stroud Ltd; Blackwell Scientific Publications Ltd; Mr D. Bourne; A.E. Dean and Co. Ltd (GEC Medical Equipment Ltd); Elema-Schonander; Mr R.F. Farr; Mr W. Herstel; International General Electric Co. of New York; Machlett X-ray Tubes (Great Britain) Ltd (GEC Medical Equipment Ltd);

Marconi Instruments Ltd; Mr G. Mountain; N.V. Optische Industrie; *Radiography*, the Journal of the Society of Radiographers; Sierex Ltd; The Technical Press Ltd; Watson and Sons (Electro-Medical) Ltd (GEC Medical Equipment Ltd).

Our colleague Mr D.S. Wilkinson took the photograph (Plate 12.2) of the handswitch of an AOT film changer, and we are grateful for his practical help.

Extracts in Chapter 5 from the British Standard Specifications for Composite Units of Switches and Fuses (British Standard 2510:1954) and for Heavy Duty Composite Units of Air-Break Switches and Fuses (British Standard 3185:1959) are reproduced by kind permission of the British Standards Institution, 2 Park Street, London W1Y 4AA, from whom copies of the complete Standard may be obtained.

Finally we would like once more to thank Mr Per Saugman of Blackwell Science who, in telling us that he would publish this book, allowed us the self-indulgence of writing it.

1970                                                    D.N.C.
                                                      M.O.C.

# Preface to the Fourth Edition

Radiographers' estimates of the importance of 'equipment' tend to change, as time passes. Aware of this, the compilers of this fourth edition of *Equipment for Student Radiographers* have studied current attitudes and priorities, in an attempt to produce a book relevant to today's needs. Before progressing to the actual text, readers are invited to spend a few minutes considering the underlying rationale.

In the early years following Röntgen's discovery of X-rays, radiographers commonly knew in detail how their X-ray equipment worked. In many instances they had built their own and, indeed, an interest in electrical apparatus alone, had led them into this new sphere. Such pioneers were joined by colleagues whose basic interests were centred elsewhere – on patient care or the anatomical and pathological aspects of the work. An academic examination system soon enforced an interest in equipment on these radiographers too, however, as part of their route to a professional qualification.

At a time when radiographers had virtually no-one else to turn to when faulty equipment needed repair, an extensive study of electrical circuitry and mechanical principles was obviously relevant. As X-ray equipment firms became established, however, and hospital installations more numerous and diverse, responsibility for electromechanical maintenance was taken over by separately trained staff. Thus the relevance of 'equipment' as it had been previously perceived, weakened in the minds of most radiographers. Yet, as operators of the equipment, they still needed a thorough comprehension of physical principles so that their work could be safe and accurate, and make best use of the equipment's capabilities. This need remains valid today even though its importance – to student radiographers, at least – may have tended to be concealed beneath overprolonged attention to irrelevancies of equipment construction.

Commercial competition, developing technology and the general influence of 'fashion' then led to the streamlining and sophistication of X-ray equipment. Unfortunately, this began to conceal the landmarks on which radiographers previously relied, as links between theory and reality. Today, progressive automation of principal functions is further widening this gulf. Modern electronic innovations are now responsible for the paradox that equipment is easier than ever to operate but more difficult than ever to understand.

During recent years, a further important factor has risen to prominence. Quality assurance, observed for many years, in many places, as an essential feature of professional practice, has now become the subject of legislation, demanding mandatory attention. As operators of expensive, high voltage equipment, exposing members of the public to ionizing radiation, radiographers carry a heavy responsibility. For the safety of their patients, themselves and fellow staff, and for economic reasons, a guarantee is needed that radiographers' skill is being complemented by their equipment's functional reliability.

Another basic fact has become more apparent during recent times. It seems too obvious to state that, 'an X-ray department is fitted with equipment which will enable it to carry out its duties'. Years ago, the situation was indeed simple: patients were X-rayed with the X-ray equipment available – the mainstay of every department being its large proportion of 'general rooms'. As technology, both electronic and surgical, has developed, however, general-purpose designs have given way to specialization. 'Dedicated' equipment has been conceived to perform specific examinations with increased accuracy and efficiency. Thus, an imaging department's complement of equipment has become more strongly related to the profile of examinations it has been called upon to perform. In recent years, dramatic changes in work profile have taken place in all but the smallest X-ray departments.

Specialization is characterized by loss of flexibility, however, and – to complicate the situation – a large number of examinations now no longer involve the use of X-rays, at all. (Indeed, the traditional label 'X-ray department' has been discarded by most hospitals, in favour of a more accurate title recognizing the breadth of diagnostic imaging techniques.) Significant innovations are procedures using ultrasound, radionuclides and magnetic resonance as the imaging modalities and computer-generated, rather than direct, image formation. A radiographer's learning cannot, therefore, now be confined to X-ray equipment: other diagnostic imaging methods need to be included, and expansion of this Fourth Edition's coverage reflects this greater need.

A consequence of stronger links between techniques and equipment is vulnerability to shifting fashion: a masterpiece of dedicated equipment becomes redundant when its particular application fades from the current range of diagnostic procedures. A textbook which attempts to be fully comprehensive and cumulative, describing every type of diagnostic imaging equipment, would nowadays be a truly massive volume. A considerable amount of editing has therefore been exercised in the following text, compared with its predecessor. Descriptions of equipment which now tends to be obsolete have been excluded except where a brief account serves as a useful background to comprehension. The term 'comprehension' is significant. It is not, and never has been, enough for a radiographer simply to remember that the X-ray tube has an anode or that a grid has lines. Memorized knowledge is lost as easily as it is gained. The real need is for comprehension and intelligent appreciation of physical principles which have a direct bearing on safe, accurate and efficient use of equipment. Where background physics is required, some readers will already be familiar with the relevant facts and principles. Others, however, may be less certain. In order to cover this need, therefore, supporting explanations are incorporated where appropriate.

Following the example – indeed, one might say, the tradition – set by Muriel and Noreen Chesney, the writers of this new edition have tried to match the scope, depth and balance of this book to the requirements of student radiographers. It is our hope that students will look on the equipment which surrounds them in their clinical departments with interest: neither being apathetic nor, in any real sense, afraid of it. The chapters of this book end with suggested *Follow-up* material to make their book learning come alive. In return, it is hoped that this particular text can shed some light on the occasional puzzles encountered in clinical practice. An enquiring attitude can enrich the experience of being a student radiographer – and be evident in enhanced care of and service to the patient.

It is recognized, of course, that today's students are tomorrow's qualified staff, with aspirations to higher qualifications and promotion. But the greater responsibilities of evaluating and choosing equipment are built on foundations laid during student days. It is hoped that this book, with its limitations (since it is only a book), can make a contribution to each reader's future career.

*Peter Carter*
Sheffield, 1993

# Acknowledgements

Compilation of this new edition of *Chesneys' Equipment for Student Radiographers*, has involved more work than may be apparent to the reader. I would like, therefore, to record my gratitude to those colleagues, without whom this work would not have been completed. I am grateful particularly to Audrey Paterson and Mike Thornton, for their chapters which give this new edition its particular (and, I believe, future) significance. I must also record my thanks to John Pirrie, Andrew Hyatt and Andrew Milne, for their written contributions and for critical comments on the text's overall structure.

X-ray equipment is continually being outdated by its own developments; today's routine is tomorrow's history. I am indebted, therefore, to Tony Doherty of International General Electric Medical Systems Ltd; to Andrew Jeffery, of Siemens plc; and Norman Clarke of Philips Medical Systems for their generous help, and to their respective companies for permission to reproduce photographs and diagrams of their equipment. Thanks are also due to Anita Littlechild of Philips Medical Systems, to David Sanders of Siemens plc and to Valerie Head, for providing photographs and diagrams.

These companies have contributed to the whole book, but particular thanks for help with Chapter 17 are offered to Christine Solimanpour, formerly of Picker International Ltd, and Sandie Jewell of IGE Medical Systems for assistance in collecting and preparing much of the technical data in this chapter and to Lister Bestcare for providing the photograph of the MR unit in clinical use. Help with Chapter 17 must also be acknowledged from Janice Ward, the radiographers and the Clinical Director of the MR Unit at St James's University Hospital, Leeds. They have given valuable support by both allowing observation of their clinical procedures and providing MR images.

Help in the compilation of Chapter 16 is acknowledged again from Philips, Siemens and IGE and from Acuson Limited, Advanced Technology Laboratories UK Ltd, Aloka Co Ltd, Dornier Medical Systems (UK), Kretztechnik (UK) Ltd, Diasonics Sonotron and Toshiba Medical Systems Ltd.

I would like to express my sincerest gratitude to the following:

Firstly, the staff of Blackwell Science, particularly Lisa Field,

Sue Moore, Peter Saugman and Richard Miles – who have shown a patience in face of delay after delay, which should be stamped on every page of this book.

Secondly, readers should know that even this delayed publication would not have been possible without the support and co-operation I have received from my wife, Sheila, and children, Helen and Nicholas.

Thirdly, I must record my respect for the fact that Muriel and Noreen Chesney not only wrote this book originally, but then took it through three editions. The perpetuation of their name in the title of this Fourth Edition is a pleasure rather than a duty.

Peter Carter
Sheffield 1993

# Part One
# The X-Ray Tube

Although quite complex, the X-ray tube has been chosen as the starting point of this revised text because of its central importance to radiographic and fluoroscopic equipment. Coverage – a suggested learning path – is in six sections:

1.1 *X-ray production* – a description of the tube's main function.
1.2 *Electrical and radiation safety* – an outline of how X-ray production can be achieved without danger to the operator or the patient.
1.3 *Focal spot size* – a look at how tube operation can affect image unsharpness.
1.4 *The problem of heat* – a consideration of its influence on tube design.
1.5 *X-ray tube construction and operation* – a detailed account of the tube components and how they together form both stationary anode and rotating anode tubes.
1.6 *Care of the X-ray tube* – a summary of how the user can delay or even prevent tube breakdown.

# Chapter 1
# The X-Ray Tube

## 1.1 X-ray production

Before learning about X-ray tube design and operation, it is essential to know the physical principle of X-ray production: X-rays are produced *when high-speed electrons suddenly undergo a change in direction.*

Although we usually say that an X-ray tube 'produces' X-rays, it is helpful to realize that this 'production' is really a process of *conversion*: an X-ray tube converts its input of electrical energy into an output of X-ray energy.

In order to achieve this energy conversion, we find that an X-ray tube provides:

(1) A supply of electrons which are free to move.
(2) A means of getting these electrons to travel at high speed.
(3) A force which will cause these fast-moving electrons suddenly to change direction.

These are provided as follows.

### Production of free electrons

The source of electrons is a **filament**, heated by an electric current. The current increases the vibration of atoms within the filament so much that it emits heat and light. These are energy forms converted from the energy of electrons flowing through the filament.

So much heat energy is acquired by the atoms that some of their electrons (outer, negatively-charged particles) can break free and temporarily leave the filament's surface. This phenomenon is known as thermionic emission. The rate at which electrons are emitted rises with the filament's temperature.

When a body loses electrons, it becomes positively charged. This happens to the filament when thermionic emission occurs. Loss of electrons is therefore followed by re-attraction. Thus, a simultaneous emission/re-attraction cycle is established. As the electrons cycle round, they form a negatively-charged cloud, or *space charge*, close to the filament.

## *The electrons' acceleration to a high speed*

The filament, forming part of the X-ray tube's **cathode**, is situated a short distance away from the **anode**. The electrons forming the space charge are dramatically affected when an X-ray exposure is made. When the exposure button is pressed, a high electrical potential difference is applied across the tube: the anode becomes strongly positive and the cathode strongly negative. Because they are negatively charged, the space charge electrons each acquire a large measure of potential energy: the anode exerts a strong attraction, while the cathode exerts a strong repulsion. Then immediately, because they are free to move, the electrons set off towards the anode. As they travel, their potential energy is converted into kinetic energy, so that they travel faster and faster. By the time they reach the anode, the electrons have accelerated to a very high speed – that is, they have acquired a large amount of kinetic energy.

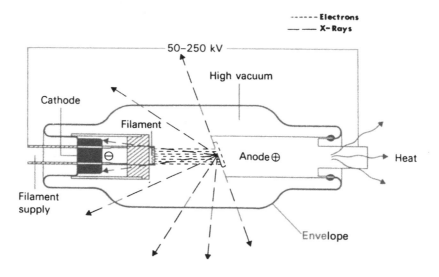

**Fig. 1.1** A fixed anode X-ray tube. Electrons travelling from cathode to anode have some of their kinetic energy converted into X-rays. Note that X-rays are emitted from the target in all directions. (*By courtesy of IGE Medical Systems.*)

It is possible for the electrons to be emitted freely from the filament and to travel unimpeded across to the anode, because they are in a **vacuum**. This condition exists because both cathode and anode are sealed into an evacuated glass **envelope**.

## *The electrons' sudden change of direction*

Instead of travelling to every part of the anode, the electrons are forced to form a narrowing beam, converging on a specific part of the anode, the

**target**. This is achieved by taking advantage of the electrons' negative charge. The filament is recessed in a **focusing cup** which, being part of the cathode, is at a high negative potential. The focusing cup therefore repels the electrons – not simply towards the anode but into a convergent beam, directed precisely at the target.

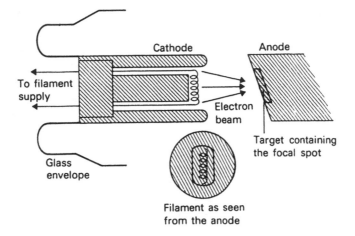

**Fig. 1.2** Electron beam focusing. The filament is recessed within a focusing cup. The cup's negative potential repels the electrons into forming a convergent beam directed towards the target.

Being negatively charged, electrons tend to be attracted towards any point at positive potential. The natural location of an electron is within an atom, held by a force of attraction towards the atomic nucleus. This attractive force is employed for the purpose of producing X-rays. The target is usually made of **tungsten**, an element with an atomic number of 74: in other words, there is a positive charge of 74 units on the nucleus of every tungsten atom. The target's nuclei can therefore exert strong, positive, attractive forces on the electrons passing through, on their way from the filament. These are the forces responsible for suddenly changing the electrons' direction of travel.

(It may be apparent that only one of these three conditions – the force which makes the high speed electrons suddenly change direction – is actually provided by the tube alone. The other two (energy, both to heat the filament and accelerate the free electrons) come from the X-ray generator which supplies the tube.)

## Energy conversion into X-rays

There are actually two ways in which X-rays may be produced when high-speed electrons bombard the X-ray tube's target. Under laboratory conditions, it is possible to distinguish these two types from each other, but for most clinical purposes they are identical.

### Production of Braking Radiation (or bremsstrahlung)

When they reach the target, only a minority of the electrons from the filament – perhaps 5% – will pass close enough to a nuclei of target atoms to experience a force of attraction. This important minority are responsible for most of the X-ray production. As they are momentarily drawn towards an orbital path around a nucleus, the sudden change in direction converts some of their kinetic energy into a quantity of X-ray energy.

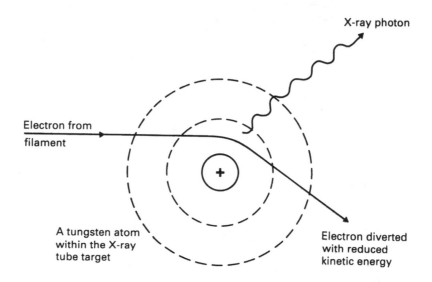

**Fig. 1.3** Production of bremsstrahlung (*braking X-rays*). Some of the electrons bombarding the target pass close enough to its atoms' nuclei to be attracted away from their original paths. The sudden change in direction converts kinetic into X-ray energy. As a result of these conversions, the electrons slow down.

The quantity produced by a single conversion event is known as an X-ray **photon**. The loss of kinetic energy causes the electrons to slow down – a fact which led to X-rays produced in this manner becoming known as: *braking radiation* (or, in German, the native language of Wilhelm Röntgen, the discoverer of X-rays, *bremsstrahlung*).

The relatively strong attraction which can be exerted on an electron by the nucleus of a high atomic number element tends to make energy conversions into X-rays more efficient than they would be with a lower atomic number. The exact value of a bremsstrahlung photon's energy, however, is unpredictable: it depends on chance – ranging from a 100% conversion of the electron's kinetic energy, down to a small, indeterminate value at the lower limits of detection.

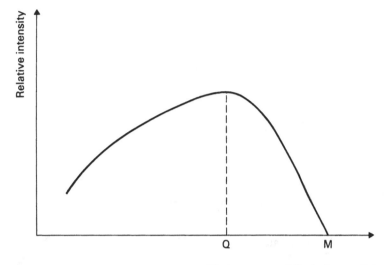

**Fig. 1.4** A continuous X-ray spectrum. This shows the range of bremsstrahlung photon energies present in an X-ray beam. Relative intensities indicate how commonly the various photon energies are present within the beam. The most commonly occurring or modal photon energy, *Q*, is an indicator of the beam's quality (penetrating power). The intensities of photon energies above *Q* become less as the likelihood of filament electrons passing closer to target nuclei becomes less. A 100% conversion produces the maximum photon energy, *M*, (where photon energy in keV numerically equals the peak kilovoltage across the X-ray tube). The relative rarity of this event is shown by its low intensity. The growth of intensities, from the lowest photon energy up to *Q*, demonstrates the photons' increasing ability to penetrate the filtration layers lying in the path of the X-ray beam.

## Production of characteristic X-rays

The other process by which X-rays are produced also involves a small minority of the electrons which bombard the target. When they reach the tube target, some of them collide with electrons orbiting the nuclei of target atoms. If an electron from the filament has more energy than the orbiting electron with which it collides, the collision removes this electron from its orbit. The collision thus creates a vacancy. This is filled immediately: an electron from a shell further out from the nucleus travels quickly inwards and swings into this inner orbital path. This electron gains its speed by having its potential energy converted into kinetic energy. The sudden change of direction when it enters its new orbit results in a further conversion – into an X-ray photon. The photons produced by this process have accurately measurable values: they equal the differences in electron binding energies between

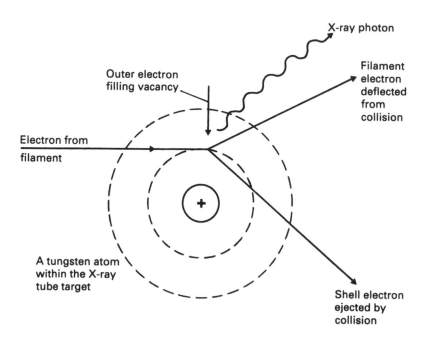

**Fig. 1.5** Production of characteristic X-ray photons. Some electrons from the filament collide with target electrons. If its kinetic energy is greater than the binding energy, a filament electron can displace a target electron, to create a vacancy. The filling of such a vacancy, by an electron from an outer shell, is accompanied by energy conversion into an X-ray photon.

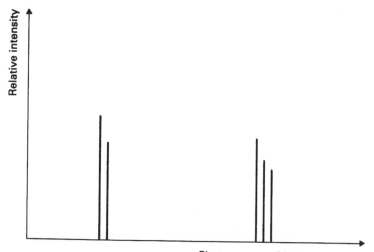

**Fig. 1.6** Line spectra. Characteristic X-ray photons have exact values, equal to the differences between the binding energies of shells involved in vacancy-filling electron transitions.

(1)  The inner shell in which the vacancy is created and then filled, and
(2)  The outer shell from which the electron travels to fill the vacancy.

Shell binding energies are known characteristics, unique to each element. For this reason, X-rays produced by these vacancy filling transitions are termed *characteristic* X-rays.

Again, the relatively high atomic number of the target material is relevant. The electron binding energy of a given shell is defined as the energy required to remove an electron from that shell. Such removal requires the binding force exerted by the nucleus (positive attracting negative) to be overcome. The strength of this force increases with the element's atomic number – a higher value indicating a more strongly positive nucleus. As the atomic number increases, so does an element's binding energies and, relevantly, the differences between them. Thus, the characteristic X-ray photons emitted from a target have higher energies when the target material has a higher atomic number.

## 1.2  Electrical and radiation safety

Due to the very high voltages at which it operates, even more insulation is required in an X-ray tube than in an everyday domestic appliance. The flexible cables which conduct high voltage supplies to and from the tube are heavily insulated with rubber or plastic. Their connections into the tube via the cable ports continue this insulation with ceramic and other rigid insulating materials. Inside the tube itself, the space between the glass insert and the outer **housing** is completely filled with a special type of insulating **oil**.

At these very high voltages, safety is not left solely to insulation. A secondary reinforcement is provided, termed **shockproofing**. This takes the form of a metallic shield, external to the insulation, at earth (zero) potential. The shield is formed by

(1)  The tube housing,
(2)  An outer metallic sheath covering the whole length of the high voltage (*high tension*) cables, and
(3)  The tank containing the source of the high voltage, the high tension transformer.

If the insulation fails, electric charge from the internal conductors can flow safely to earth via this surrounding shield, instead of via a person who chances to touch this equipment. The term **shockproofed** is thus explained.

X-rays are emitted from the tube target *in all directions*. Because of the biological dangers involved in the use of X-rays, it is important that the X-ray beam should only emerge from the tube through the window. The inside of the tube housing is therefore lined with sheet lead. This absorbs the X-rays so efficiently that only a very small rate of leakage occurs.

## 1.3  Focal spot size

Electron bombardment of the target has been described, so far without mention of target size, other than a mention that it is *small*. The reason why it should be small is found in the facts that

(1)  It is the source of the X-ray beam, and
(2)  The X-ray beam is used (for diagnostic purposes) to produce images.

### X-ray penumbra

Radiographic images are compiled from X-ray shadows. The simplest imaginable situation would be where shadows are cast within a radiation beam coming from a single point source. Such an arrangement is possible with visible light. Within a cine or slide projector, an optical system focuses light from a lamp so that it appears to come from a point source. It can then pass through a small transparent image on a film, to display it as a large image, sharply on a distant screen.

Unfortunately, this arrangement cannot be achieved in radiographic imaging. Unlike visible light, X-rays cannot be focused; they have to be used 'as they come' – and the size of their source cannot, therefore, be as small as an infinitely small point. The effect of the source's finite size is that every X-ray shadow is surrounded by a zone of partial shadow, termed the **penumbra**. Penumbra becomes visible as image unsharpness. To distinguish it from other causes (movement blur, for example) the effect of penumbra is usually termed **geometric unsharpness**.

To restrict geometric unsharpness, an X-ray tube is designed to have a small radiation source area. One design feature, already mentioned, is the electron beam focusing arrangement: the filament is recessed within a focusing cup which is at a high, repelling, negative potential. So, despite being emitted from a filament of some size, the electrons converge to bombard a much smaller area.

### Angulation of the target

The target of an X-ray tube is set at an angle which allows both free access for the approaching electron beam and a suitably wide exit path for the emerging X-rays. This angulation also forms a clever compromise between

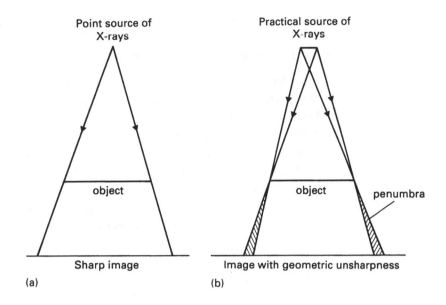

**Fig. 1.7** Penumbra. A practical X-ray source is a volume within the anode (having length, width and depth) rather than a theoretical point source. It acts as a cluster of point sources, each casting its own shadow of the radiographic object. Most of these separate shadows overlap to form a whole image but there are peripheral, incomplete shadows (penumbra) which do not overlap, thus giving the image an unsharp appearance. To distinguish this from other causes, the term **geometric unsharpness** is used.

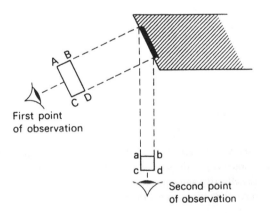

**Fig. 1.8** The line focus principle. Angulation of the anode face results in an oblong bombarded target surface (relatively large, for efficient heat spread) which presents a foreshortened, square appearance (small, to restrict penumbra) from the perspective of the central X-ray.

(1) The physical reality of a bombarded area which, although small, still has some size and

(2) The need for a radiation source which is even smaller.

The target bombarded by filament electrons actually has an oblong area. Viewed from the perspective of the *central X-ray*, however, (along the middle of the beam which emerges from the tube), it is foreshortened to a square. This is the area from which the X-ray beam appears to come; it determines the penumbra size and the resulting image unsharpness. It is known as either the **apparent** or **effective focal area**. Perhaps more commonly and simply, it is known as the X-ray tube's **focal spot**. To distinguish it from its foreshortened version, the oblong area bombarded by electrons is known as the **actual** or **true focal area**.

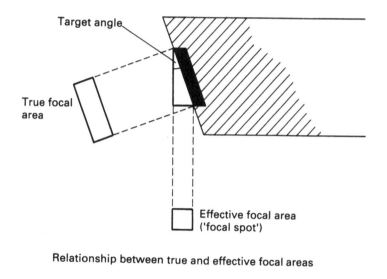

Relationship between true and effective focal areas

$$\text{Sine of target angle} = \frac{\text{opposite}}{\text{hypotenuse}}$$

$$= \frac{\text{EFA}}{\text{TFA}}$$

**Fig. 1.9** Relationship between true and effective focal areas. This relationship is determined by the target (anode) angle: the sine of the angle (opposite/hypotenuse) is the ratio between the *lengths* of the effective and true focal areas. Since these areas share a common *width*, the sine also measures the ratio between their areas.

Efforts to reduce the true focal area, by more intense focusing of the electron beam, are limited due to an effect of electron bombardment described in the next section.

## 1.4 The problem of heat

So far, X-ray production has been portrayed as a fairly simple affair: electrons are produced by the tube filament and then made to bombard the target. Thus, X-rays are produced! Students may suspect – and would be correct in doing so – that matters are not quite so simple.

The problem which surrounds the production of X-rays is common in energy conversion equipment. A simple light bulb and a car engine provide two instances: energy conversion is not only into the desired form (light energy, kinetic energy); heat is produced, as well.

It has been mentioned that only a minority of the electrons which bombard the target have their energy converted into X-rays. The majority of the electrons lose their kinetic energy gradually, during a series of collisions with the target atoms. These begin to vibrate at increased rates, causing the target temperature to rise.

The commonest material used for target construction is the element tungsten. This has the highest melting point of all the known metallic elements (a reason why it is chosen). Even so, steps must be taken, by careful design and operation, to minimize the temperature rise which accompanies X-ray production. Otherwise, thermal damage may be caused which could end the tube's working life or, at least, reduce its efficiency.

The risk of damage can be limited if attention is given to four issues:

(1) Minimizing the quantity of heat produced.
(2) Minimizing the rate at which heat is produced.
(3) Increasing the area bombarded by the electrons, to limit the temperature rise produced by a given quantity of heat.
(4) Providing efficient cooling pathways for heat to leave the bombarded area and spread out to surrounding parts of the tube.

These will now be considered.

### (1) Minimizing the quantity of heat produced

Heat is formed at the tube target by conversion of kinetic energy possessed by electrons accelerated across from the filament. The quantity of kinetic energy is determined by three factors:

(a) The rate at which electrons bombard the target.
(b) The average kinetic energy possessed by the electrons.
(c) The duration of the bombardment.

Expressed in another way, these factors are:

(a) The electric **current** through the tube (usually measured in milliamperes (mA)).

(b) The electrical **potential difference**, the kilovoltage (kV), applied across the tube.

(c) The X-ray exposure **time** (in seconds or milliseconds).

These three factors – mA, kV and time – are selected by a radiographer before, or automatically determined during every radiographic exposure. Their function is to produce a certain quantity and quality of X-ray energy, in order to form an image.

The amount of heat produced during an exposure cannot be changed without an alteration also occurring in the quantity of X-ray energy produced; one accompanies the other. The only methods of lessening the quantity of heat, therefore, are those which, by increasing the efficiency of image formation, reduce the quantity of X-ray energy needed for an exposure. Examples include the use of faster (more sensitive) image recording materials.

## *(2) Minimizing the rate at which heat is produced*

If the rate of heat production is restricted, an opportunity is created to cool the tube target, actually during its bombardment. This simultaneous loss of heat increases the tube target's capacity for safely accepting heat, and so lessens the risk of thermal damage.

The direct link between heat and X-ray production must be borne in mind, however, if a reduction is sought in the rate of heat production. This rate can easily be restricted if the tube's operator is happy to accept a proportionately lower rate of X-ray production. In diagnostic radiography, this may not always be the case; sharp images have to be produced, of objects which have the potential to move. Movement during the exposure and the image blurring it can cause, can best be limited if exposure times are kept short.

To produce a required quantity of X-ray energy, the exposure time can be shortened only if the rate of production is increased – which inevitably increases the rate of heat production. This matter – which concerns the manner in which a tube is used, rather then how it is constructed – is the subject of safety restrictions imposed by X-ray tube manufacturers, as a tube's **rating**. This will be discussed later in the chapter.

## *(3) Increasing the area bombarded by the electrons*

The temperature rise of any heated body, created by a given quantity of heat, is inversely related to its thermal capacity. In the case of an X-ray tube, if the target is small, the temperature rise caused by an X-ray exposure will be relatively high. If the target is large, the rise will be less. Enlargement of the target, however, would simply aggravate another problem. As already described, the source of the X-ray beam – or, at least, its apparent (effective) size – should be small, to minimize penumbra and subsequent geometric unsharpness of the image. Ideally, therefore, any effort to increase the area bombarded by electrons must be achieved without increasing the area from which the X-ray beam appears to come.

### The anode or target angle

Angulation of the target has already been mentioned. It enables a compromise to be achieved between these conflicting demands for a large heated area, and a small radiation source area. More attention can now be given to the exact angle at which the target is set.

The angle precisely controls the ratio between the heated area and the area responsible for penumbra. In other words, it controls the *ratio* between true and effective focal areas. The trigonometrical sine of the target angle (opposite/hypoteneuse) is the side length of the (square) effective focal area divided by the length of the (oblong) true focal area. Since both these areas have a common width, it is thus also the ratio between the areas themselves.

Reduction of this angle therefore enhances the relationship: the steeper the angle, the larger the heated area and the smaller the X-ray source. The angle cannot be reduced indefinitely, however. As it approaches zero, a practical problem arises. The sloping face of the target forms a limiting boundary to the edge of the useful beam. X-rays directed behind this boundary are wholly absorbed within the anode.

### The *anode heel* effect

Absorption of X-rays within the anode itself potentially raises another problem. Because it tends to be taken from the periphery of the whole emission from the target, the useful beam suffers from an uneven intensity. Measured along the anode–cathode axis, the radiation forming the X-ray field at its *cathode side* may be more intense than across at the *anode side*, where the radiation has emerged from the target at a near-grazing angle.

This *anode heel* effect may have no practical significance, particularly if field size is small. When the whole width of the beam is used, however, its intensity variation may cause a detectable contrast in image density, from one end to the other.

### Principle of the rotating anode

So far, the simplest type of X-ray tube has been described, which has a stationary or fixed anode. The most significant advance in diagnostic X-ray tube design was achieved with the invention of the rotating anode. Its inventors cleverly analysed the conflict between thermal capacity and penumbra, and realized that the areas

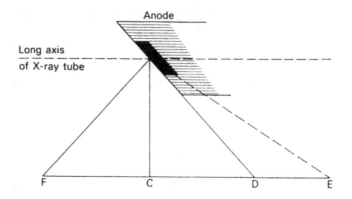

**Fig. 1.10** *Anode heel* variation of X-ray intensity. Intensity at F is greater than at C, which itself is greater than at D. Beyond D – for example, at E – there is no significant radiation, due to absorption within the anode.

(1) Heated by electron bombardment and
(2) Within which X-rays are produced

need not be identical. They also suggested and proved that X-ray production stays unaffected when electrons bombard a moving area.

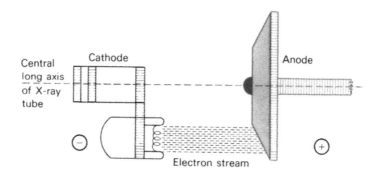
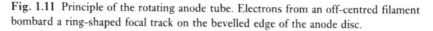

**Fig. 1.11** Principle of the rotating anode tube. Electrons from an off-centred filament bombard a ring-shaped focal track on the bevelled edge of the anode disc.

Within a rotating anode tube, the area bombarded by electrons, instead of being a small, rectangular source, identical to the X-ray source, is a broad, ring-shaped focal track. Rotation of this track continuously carries the recently heated area out of the way of the oncoming electrons, presenting to them a fresh, cooler area.

Almost all the X-ray tubes in use in imaging departments have rotating anodes. They have displaced the fixed anode tube from clinical use, because of the *much higher rate of X-ray production* which they can achieve. Consequent benefits are found in short exposure times, and images *unaffected by movement blur*.

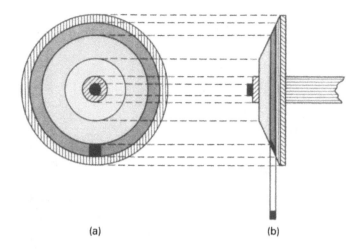

(a)             (b)

**Fig. 1.12** A conventional rotating anode disc. (a) Face view; (b) In profile. While electrons still (as with a fixed anode) bombard a small, rectangular area, the heat caused by conversion of their energy is spread around a much larger area, the disc's focal track.

### *(4) Providing efficient cooling pathways*

If left for long enough, any heated body will eventually cool down. X-ray tubes, however, require something which is more immediate and efficient. From its source, where electron bombardment occurs, the heat generated alongside X-ray production must be led along pathways, as quickly as possible, to restrict the damaging effects of a temperature rise.

The methods by which fixed and rotating anodes are cooled, are distinctly different – and will be described as integral features of their whole design.

## 1.5. X-ray tube construction and operation

### *The fixed anode tube*

#### Cathode
The cathode, the electrode which operates at a high negative potential, has three parts:

(1) A large, basic structure or **body** is sealed into the glass envelope. It encloses the wires which carry the electrical connections and it extends forwards (towards the anode) to support:
(2) The **focusing cup**, within which is mounted
(3) The **filament**.

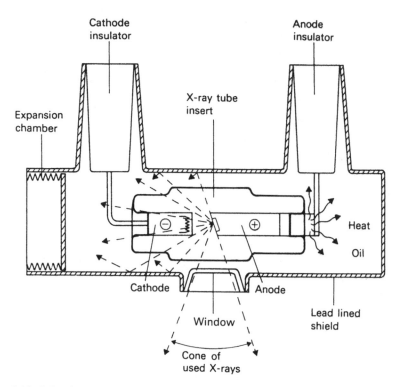

**Fig. 1.13** A fixed anode X-ray tube: insert and housing. (*By courtesy of IGE Medical Systems.*)

*Focusing cup*

This is an elongated, deep and open structure. It may have a curved or square profile. Its electrical connection is to the highly negative output (typically in the range from minus 30 kV to minus 60 kV) from the X-ray generator. This strong negative potential exerts a repelling force on the electrons emitted from the filament. They thus leave the cathode as an ordered, converging beam, directed precisely onto the target area of the anode. The shape of the focusing cup and the position of the filament are very precisely calculated and manufactured. This ensures the accuracy of the target size (true focal area). Focusing cups are usually made of either nickel or stainless steel.

In some specialized X-ray tubes, the negative potential applied to the focusing cup can be varied. The effects of variation are to alter the degree of electron beam convergence, thus varying the focal spot size, and, when a large, *blocking* potential is applied, to prevent emission altogether. This effect may be employed to switch X-ray exposures on and off.

*Filament*

The filament is in the form of a linear spiral. It is mounted within the focusing cup but has its own distinct electrical supply. One end of the filament is usually connected to the focusing cup and is therefore at its same potential, but the other end is electrically insulated from the focusing cup. A low voltage is applied across the filament, from the filament transformer within the X-ray generator.

The filament is made of tungsten. This element is widely used in filament construction, not only for X-ray tubes. Its properties include:

(1) A very high melting point – an obviously important need for a filament which has to operate at high temperatures. In fact, at 3300°C tungsten has the highest melting point of any metallic element.
(2) Favourable manufacturing properties: it is said to be **ductile** – that is, it can be drawn out into a fine wire; retaining its shape even when hot.
(3) It is a ready emitter of electrons: it is said to have a low **work function** – that is, a relatively low amount of energy can release electrons from its atoms. Moreover, the rate of release can be accurately controlled – an important factor in achieving a precise rate of X-ray production.
(4) Tungsten is said to produce a low **vapour pressure**; that is, it vaporizes at a relatively low rate, despite being heated to high temperatures. This is important for achieving a reasonably long filament life. Vaporization causes a filament to become thinner, as atoms are lost from its surface. Thinning interferes with the filament's correct functioning and may eventually cause it to break.

## Anode

The anode of a fixed anode tube is relatively simple: a rectangular tungsten target is embedded in the sloping surface of a copper cylinder. An obvious function of the copper cylinder is to act as a support for the target, to hold it accurately in the required position. As an electrical conductor, it easily allows the flow of electrons from the target and into the continuing electrical circuit.

It has another extremely important function: it provides a cooling pathway which conducts heat from the target, restricting its temperature rise.

The remote end of the cylinder, furthest from the target, lies outside the tube insert, surrounded by oil. As well as acting as an electrical insulator, the oil serves to convect heat from the central, heated parts of the tube to its outer housing. Thus the remote end of the copper cylinder is at a relatively low temperature, compared with the target. When heat is produced at the target, during an X-ray exposure, a temperature gradient is established. Heat always travels from a hotter place to a cooler place. In this case, heat travels from the target by conduction along the copper anode cylinder, to its far end, immersed in oil. Within the oil, the heat then travels by convection, to the tube housing.

There is a second cooling pathway: heat can also leave the cylinder by the process of radiation, across the vacuum, to and through the glass envelope. The process of heat radiation occurs most efficiently when the source temperature is high. It thus mainly concerns the target itself and its immediate surroundings.

### Tungsten as a target material

It is coincidental that tungsten is used as a constructional material for both the filament and the target of an X-ray tube. Two properties make tungsten suitable for both purposes:

(1) Its high melting point; the target's temperature may exceed even the filament's.
(2) Its low vaporization pressure; loss of tungsten into the vacuum must be minimized from this source too.

A third property is exclusive to the role of the target:

(3) Tungsten has a relatively high atomic number, 74. An element's atomic number expresses the magnitude of the positive charge on its atoms' nuclei. It also controls the binding energies possessed by the orbiting electrons. Both of these features make tungsten a relatively efficient converter of the bombarding electrons' kinetic energy into X-ray energy (both bremsstrahlung and characteristic).

Lastly, there are suitable physical properties:

(4) Tungsten can be formed into a block with a smooth, durable surface; its expansion rate is comparable with copper's, keeping the tungsten block secure in its recess, when the anode's temperature rises.

### Envelope

The anode and cathode are sealed into an evacuated container, the envelope. To maintain electrical insulation, the electrodes must be separated by a distance in proportion to the maximum kilovoltage at which the tube is designed to operate. The envelope is usually made of a special, borosilicate glass. This is:

(1) Heat-resistant – withstanding, without cracking, the internal stresses caused by sudden temperature rise. It is very similar to the type used for ovenware.
(2) Strong – so that it holds the electrodes in their precise positions; and withstands the forces arising from having a vacuum within and oil (subject to expansion) outside.

(3) An electrical insulator. It prevents electrical conduction (discharge) between the electrode connections and the earthed housing.
(4) Radiolucent – it transmits the X-ray beam with the minimum of attenuation.

The ends of the envelope are made *re-entrant*, folded back (inside) for strength and to lengthen their conductive path. The vacuum is created to a high degree: the insert is pumped to exhaustion over a period of days, during its manufacture, before the envelope is finally sealed.

Some specialized, heavy duty tubes are built with metal envelopes. This feature has to be combined with others. For example, it conflicts with (3) above. The metal envelope incorporates insulating, ceramic fitments where the electrode connections enter the envelope. The envelope is at earth potential, to conduct away any stray electrons which deviate from the required filament–anode path. These electrons thus cannot return to the anode – where they could possibly produce extrafocal radiation – and cannot establish a charged area of the envelope, to create discharge problems.

### Inherent filtration

An X-ray tube is constructed so that the *useful beam* emerges through the window in the housing, having had its intensity reduced as little as possible. Almost always, the beam then undergoes added filtration, in the form of thin aluminium plates fixed to the outside of the tube port. The principle remains, however, that parts of the tube lying in the path of the useful beam are made as radiolucent as possible, to minimize the tube's inherent filtration.

The first layer which the beam encounters is the glass envelope wall. An area aligned with the target and the window may be ground down or moulded to a reduced thickness. This allows the beam to pass through more easily, but does not weaken the envelope's strength.

Surrounding the insert, the oil necessarily lies in the path of the useful beam and thus also contributes to the inherent filtration. This effect is lessened by closure of the window by a convex, plastic, oil-displacement cone. This protrudes into the tube cavity, reducing the thickness of the oil layer through which the useful beam has to travel, but it still allows the oil to convect through a clearance space between the cone and the envelope.

### Oil and housing

The oil which surrounds the insert acts as both an electrical insulator and a cooling convectant, carrying heat from the outer surface of the envelope to the inner wall of the tube housing. For safety, to prevent leakage, the oil is very securely sealed within the housing. This poses a potential problem because, as its temperature rises, the oil expands. If the cavity containing the oil were to be fixed and inflexible, this expansion could dangerously increase the pressure exerted both internally on the insert and externally on the seams of the housing. To overcome this problem, the wall at one end of the oil cavity is made flexible, in the form of a **bellows** device or **movable diaphragm**. By movement in and out, it can safely accommodate the fluctuating volume.

Situated directly outside the diaphragm or bellows is a **pressure-sensitive switch** which can disconnect the tube's high voltage electrical supply, if the temperature ever reaches a dangerously high value (so that the increased pressure threatens to burst the housing).

The tube housing itself is a cylinder of aluminium or mild steel, sealed at both ends. Its functions are:

(1) To contain the oil securely, without leakage, and protect the insert against damage.

Because X-rays not only form the *useful beam* but are emitted forwards from the face of the target, in all directions, a further function is:

(2) To form a protective shield against the escape of X-rays emitted in all other directions except through the window (or port). This is carefully aligned with the central ray of the useful beam.

The tube housing itself is made for strength rather than radiation protection. It meets the need for protection by having a lining of sheet lead, curved and moulded to follow the housing's contours. This lead barrier reduces the intensity of X-rays which manage to pass through it – **leakage** radiation – down to an extremely low level, permitted by protection regulations as being safe.

Surrounding the outer rim of the tube's port, the protective lining is particularly thick, to deepen the opening. This arrangement absorbs X-rays produced when stray electrons strike areas of the anode outside the target. This **extrafocal** radiation may cause image quality to deteriorate and is most effectively removed, close to its source.

The tube's housing has one further purpose:

(3) It provides electrical safety by shockproofing the tube. The housing is at earth (zero) potential through its connection to the earthed braiding which ensheaths the high voltage cables feeding into it, and also by its earthed mounting support. By this provision, safety for both patients and staff is ensured, even if there is an accidental failure of the protective insulation – for example, as a consequence of an undetected oil leak.

**Insert supports**

These structures encircle and support the tube insert, holding it firmly and accurately in its place within the tube housing. They prevent movement of the insert, so that the precise relationship of the target to the centre of the tube window is maintained.

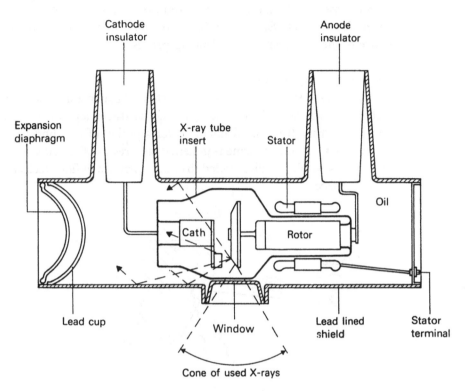

**Fig. 1.14** A rotating anode X-ray insert and housing. (*By courtesy of IGE Medical Systems.*)

## The rotating anode X-ray tube

The most radically different part of the rotating anode tube, compared with the fixed anode tube, is the anode itself. Whereas with a fixed anode, the target is both the source of X-rays and the bombarded, heated area, on a rotating anode these two are *different*. The X-ray source remains a rectangular area but the heated area is in the form of a ring or annulus, around the anode disc. This is termed the **focal track**.

Compared with a fixed anode, this design provides a greatly increased area within which heat may be produced and from which heat may more efficiently leave. The rotating anode is thus able to tolerate much higher rates of heat production than a fixed anode – and, therefore, much higher, safer rates of X-ray production.

### Anode disc

This typically has a diameter of 100 or 120 mm. Its surface facing the cathode has a sloping, bevelled edge, around which lies the focal track. The disc is mounted on a stem which arises from the rotor. This whole assembly rotates at rates which may exceed 10 000 revolutions per minute. The stresses imposed by the speeds involved require the assembly to be perfectly balanced. The reverse face of the disc may show some concave marks, as evidence of the manufacturer's balancing process.

### Focal track composition

Years ago, discs were made wholly of tungsten. On such a disc, when new, the focal track was only identifiable by being the area in alignment with the stream of electrons from the filament. After a period of use, however, the surface of the focal track became roughened, as a result of repeated heating. Inner tensions within the disc tended to create a pattern of fine cracks on the tungsten surface.

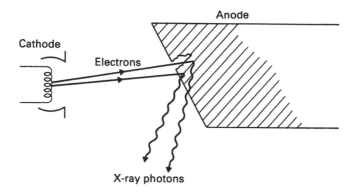

**Fig. 1.15** Effect of target surface pitting. Roughening of the target surface, due to cumulative effects of heat stress, creates **pitting**, the formation of small crevices into which electrons from the filament may enter. X-ray photons so produced have a greater thickness of anode substance to penetrate before they emerge from its surface. This reduces the beam intensity, compared with the output from a new, smooth target surface.

The practical, radiographic effect of thermal damage to the focal track is a reduction in the intensity of the X-ray beam. Photons produced below the anode surface have a thickness of superficial metal to penetrate before emerging to contribute to the useful beam. A smooth focal track limits this effect. A roughened surface enhances it: fissures are formed which electrons from the filament can enter, to produce X-ray photons deeper below the surface than in an undamaged anode. The absorption by superficial layers is thus enhanced. Compensatory increases in tube kilovoltage, current or exposure time – to maintain radiographic image densities despite this focal track deterioration – only aggravate the condition: even more heat is produced, in proportion to the X-ray output. The tube is then into its process of ageing towards eventual failure. On economic grounds, as well as concern for image quality, this underlines the need for X-ray tubes to be used carefully, so that overheating is avoided.

X-ray tube manufacturers have reduced the anode disc's susceptibility to this effect by alloying tungsten with another metal, rhenium. A modern disc usually has a focal track composed of a **90% tungsten/10% rhenium alloy**. The student may wonder whether inclusion of another element can weaken the focal track's ability to produce X-rays. While rhenium's melting point is lower than tungsten's, its atomic number is actually higher – 75, compared with 74 – so energy conversion efficiency is maintained. Modern discs also have design features which combat the effects of internal thermal stresses. The inner and outer margins of the focal track may be marked by concave expansion grooves which can safely narrow as the heated area expands. Alternatively, some discs have radial slits which divide the circular disc area into segments. Again, these spaces can close up when expansion occurs, minimizing stresses within the metal.

The focal track cools by radiating its heat forwards across the vacuum, to the envelope wall. It also loses heat by conduction from its margins, into the mass of the anode disc. It is important, therefore, that the disc has a relatively high thermal capacity – an ability to stay at a moderate temperature, even though it holds a relatively large quantity of heat energy.

### Disc size

An obvious way to increase the disc's thermal capacity is to make it larger. Mounted on its narrow stem, however, and rotated at high speeds, the need to limit mechanical stresses has to be considered. The disc must remain stable during rotation; otherwise movement of the target may occur, with consequent effects on image quality. Even so, both the thickness and the diameter of the disc are design variables.

A widening of the disc diameter lengthens the focal track, and thus increases the area within which heat is generated. Within this increased area, there may be either a lower temperature rise from a given rate of heat production or, more usefully, a higher, safe rate of heating (and X-ray production), within the limit of a given temperature rise.

The disc's diameter and thickness both affect the mass of the disc into which heat is conducted from the focal track. A larger mass is able to absorb heat more efficiently and limit the temperature rise of the focal track. As has been mentioned, however: there are mechanical limits on the increases which can be tolerated, in both diameter and thickness.

**Table 1.1** Some significant properties of elements used in X-ray tube construction.

| Element | Use in X-ray tubes | Atomic number | Melting point (°C) | Density (kgm⁻³) | Thermal conductivity (Wm⁻¹ K⁻¹) | Specific thermal capacity (Jkg⁻¹ K⁻¹) |
|---|---|---|---|---|---|---|
| Aluminium | Beam filtration Tube housing | 13 | 660 | 2710 | 201 | 913 |
| Carbon (graphite) | Body of RA disc | 6 | 3527 | 2300 | 5 | 710 |
| Copper | RA rotor Stationary anode Electrical conductors | 29 | 1083 | 8930 | 397 | 386 |
| Lead | Radiation absorption barriers | 82 | 327 | 11340 | 35 | 126 |
| Molybdenum | Body of RA disc Target material RA disc stem | 42 | 2607 | 10200 | 137 | 251 |
| Rhenium | RA focal track, alloyed with tungsten | 75 | 3177 | 20500 | 48 | 138 |
| Tungsten | Target filament | 74 | 3300 | 19320 | 174 | 138 |

*Note:* Some data, especially those measured at extremes, are variable according to the measurement circumstances (e.g. barometric pressure). The figures shown in this table are offered to the reader principally for the purpose of identifying contrasts and comparisons – whether a value is significantly high or low.

**Disc composition**

Another method of increasing the disc's thermal capacity lies in the use of materials which (compared with the tungsten/rhenium alloy) have relatively higher specific thermal capacities and/or relatively lower densities. Such materials, notably graphite (a form of carbon) and the metal molybdenum, can absorb a greater quantity of heat energy per unit temperature rise and/or offer a larger volume (for heat absorption) per unit mass. These may be used for the main body of the disc. On account of both its high melting point and high atomic number, tungsten is retained as the principal material for the focal track.

**Anode angle**

The angle of the bevelled edge of the disc has an important influence on the width of the focal track. As previously mentioned, the anode angle controls the relationship between true and effective focal areas. For a given focal spot (effective focal area) size, a narrowing of the angle increases the focal track's area. Thus, similar to a change in disc diameter/focal track length, the maximum safe rate of X-ray production may be increased. Effects of angle reduction upon field size, already discussed, also need to be considered, however.

### Anode stem

The stem on which the disc is mounted is narrow: it has a small cross-sectional area. This design feature, while potentially lowering the anode's mechanical stability, is responsible for two important effects on disc cooling. Firstly, it *reduces the rate at which heat is conducted* along its length towards the rotation mechanism. Some rise in the rotor's temperature is inevitable but the smaller this is, the better. With a rise in temperature, metals expand. In the instance of the rotation mechanism, expansion of the moving parts tends to narrow the clearance spaces between them and increase frictional wear. In an extreme case, rotation could be impeded and the mechanism could even seize up.

Secondly, by *confining heat within the disc*, the narrow stem has the effect of sustaining the disc's high temperatures. This actually enhances the rate at which the disc cools by radiation, since this rate is strongly dependent on the temperature gradient between a body and its surroundings.

The narrow stem is put under considerable stress during exposures and it requires the use of a particularly strong metal, molybdenum.

Again, a design variation may be found in some specialized, heavy duty tubes. In the metal-ceramic tube, the anode disc is mounted on an axle which has support bearings at both ends: it passes through the disc. This gives greater stability, enabling a more massive disc to be used, rotated at higher speeds.

### Anode rotation

The anode is rotated by forming part of an induction motor. The peculiar feature of this arrangement within an X-ray tube is that its constituent parts are separated by the wall of the glass envelope. The moving rotor mechanism lies within the evacuated space inside the tube insert, while the induction coils, or **stator windings**, lie outside the insert, within the surrounding oil.

The **rotor** is a hollow copper cylinder, supporting the anode stem. It is mounted on bearings, to move freely around a central steel support or shank which, at its remote end, is sealed into the glass envelope. To minimize friction, the bearings are lubricated – with a metal, either silver or lead, not a conventional lubricant. Oil would vaporize at the working temperatures and contaminate the vacuum.

Copper is used as the rotor material because of its high conductivity, both of heat and electricity. Despite the effect of the narrow stem, some heat from the disc will reach the rotor. Once there, a rapid spread will limit the

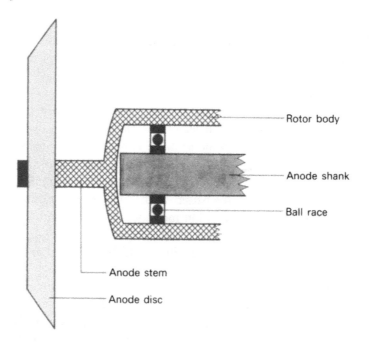

- Rotor body
- Anode shank
- Ball race
- Anode stem
- Anode disc

**Fig. 1.16** Rotating anode assembly. The disc is mounted on a relatively narrow stem, by which it is joined to the hollow, cylindrical rotor body. The rotor is free to move around the central, internal shank on a lubricated ball race.

temperature rise of the whole. Simultaneous heat loss from the rotor, to protect the bearings, is accelerated by a treatment process applied to its outer wall, during manufacture. This darkens and dulls the surface, enhancing the rate at which it loses heat by radiation. Contrasting with this, the end, *top* of the rotor is left untreated so that its shiny surface limits absorption of the heat radiated from the reverse side of the disc.

Rotation is created when alternating voltages are applied across the stator windings. The voltages are out of phase with each other, having the effect of creating a changing, rotating magnetic field. The changes in magnetic flux experienced by the rotor induce electromotive forces which cause eddy currents to flow around it. The high electrical conductivity of the copper ensures efficiency: for a given emf, the resulting current and its magnetic effect is high. The magnetic fields produced by these eddy currents react with the external fields, to create the rotational force which moves the anode. Initially, to move the rotor from its resting position, the voltages applied across the stator windings are relatively high. Once inertia has been overcome, however, and momentum established, the applied voltages are reduced to lower values. This reduction drops the rate of heat production within the windings and limits the temperature rise of the tube. A heat shield is inserted between the stator windings and the insert, as a protection between the windings and the anode.

An alternative, fluid-mounted, frictionless rotor design has been introduced in a specialized tube, but this must currently be regarded as exceptional.

### Rotational rates

While rotation of the anode disc, in principle, obviously increases the area within which heat is produced – and thus limits temperature rise – the rate at which the anode is rotated needs to be considered. The former, usual rate was approximately 3000 revolutions per minute. This struck a balance between heat-spreading benefits and the potential risks linked to rotation: mechanical wear and heat production in the stator windings. In modern practice, however, where exposure times are commonly less than the duration of one rotation, heat spread at 3000 rpm tends to be inefficient. Efficiency is improved by boosting the anode rotation rate, to spread heat more evenly around the focal track and offer an opportunity to increase the rate of heat – and X-ray – production. A rotational rate of approximately 9000 rpm may be considered as standard. This is achieved by increasing the frequency of the voltage supply to the stator windings, from 50 Hz (in the UK) to 150 Hz or 200 Hz.

High speed anode rotation can increase the risk to tube safety. There are the problems of greater wear on the moving parts, and heat production within the stator windings, plus a problem which occurs as the anode slows down. Harmful vibrations may be set up within some tube components, as the anode passes through certain frequencies – a phenomenon termed **resonance**. This problem is dealt with by the provision of a braking system to bring the anode speed quickly down, after an exposure, through and below the harmful frequencies. Since the rotor is situated within a sealed, evacuated envelope, a conventional friction braking system cannot be employed. Instead, direct voltages are applied to the stator windings, creating a stationary magnetic field which brings the rotor to a halt.

### The cathode

In most respects, the cathode of a rotating anode tube is similar to the cathode of a fixed anode tube. Two major differences may be mentioned, however. First, whereas the fixed anode tube's filament is located along the tube's central axis, the filaments of a rotating anode are off-centred, to align with the focal track around the bevelled edge of the rotating disc.

Secondly, as just hinted, while a fixed anode tube commonly has a single filament, the rotating anode tube invariably has two. These provide the tube with a facility termed **dual focus**. It is not the provision of two filaments which is remarkable, but the opportunity to use either of two dissimilar focal spots.

**Dual focus facility**

This offers to the tube operator, a choice between two sizes of focal spot. The larger is commonly referred to as the *broad* focus, and the smaller as the *fine*. In order to achieve this, there are two filaments, each within its focusing cup and independently supplied with its own voltage. The focusing cups are slightly tilted towards one another, so that the emitted electron beams bombard a common area on the anode – that is, so that the position of the focal spot does not shift with broad/fine selection.

The exact dimensions of the fine and broad focal spots are variable: tube manufacturers will supply their purchasers with focal spot sizes to match requirements. A normal range would be from 0.6 mm square, up to 1.2 mm or 1.5 mm square. Sizes outside this range would be used for special purposes. For example, a tube to be used for magnification techniques would probably need its fine focus to be as small as 0.1 mm square.

The dual focus X-ray tube acts as two tubes in one:

(1) For clinical purposes where radiography involves an *immobilized, easily penetrated* object, the operator's preference is likely to be for a *small* focal spot, to minimize penumbra and consequent *geometric unsharpness* of the image.
(2) In situations where *uncontrolled movement* of the object may be encountered, a *larger* focal spot – permitting safe production of X-rays at a higher rate, and thus *shortened exposure times* – would be preferred.

## 1.6 Care of the X-ray tube

An X-ray tube is an expensive and vulnerable piece of equipment. If damaged, it is unlikely to be repairable. There is thus a considerable responsibility on the radiographer to ensure that tubes are used carefully, to last for the full, expected term of their working lives.

Tube damage may be either physical or thermal. Physical damage is avoided simply by ensuring that the tube is never allowed to collide with any other object, and that all movement is reasonably smooth and steady. Thermal damage is minimized by

(1) Keeping the rate of heat production within the safe limits, determined by the tube manufacturer; and
(2) Ensuring, before making each exposure, that the anode can safely accept the extra heat which the exposure will bring.

Fortunately for the operator, automatic, computer-controlled safety mechanisms to protect the tube against thermal damage are a standard feature of all modern X-ray generators. They are set up in accordance with safety parameters, commonly known as the tube's rating.

## X-ray tube rating

Behind the restrictions imposed on an X-ray tube's operation, lies a concern that the rate of heat production at the tube's anode should remain within safe limits. An X-ray tube's rating is a specification of the maximum safe combinations of kV, mA and exposure time which may be used under stated circumstances, without thermal damage being caused.

### Rate of heat production

The kinetic energy possessed by each electron as it reaches the tube target is determined by the kilovoltage (kilojoules per coulomb) which caused its acceleration. The rate at which electrons arrive at the target is expressed as the tube current (coulombs or millicoulombs per second). Thus, the rate of X-ray and heat production is determined by the product of kilovoltage and current (kV × mA). This means that when the tube operator selects a value of mA or kV – in order to produce an X-ray beam of particular intensity and quality – there is a proportionate effect on the rate of heating at the tube target. So, kV and mA selection both determine the rate at which the target's temperature rises.

For every radiographic exposure, a quantity of X-radiation is required. At a given kilovoltage, this quantity is proportional to, and commonly specified by, the product of the tube current (mA) and exposure time (s). Whether the rate of production (mA) is high and the time brief, or the rate low and the time long, the quantity of X-radiation and its probable image-forming effect will be constant. The quantity of heat produced will also remain constant.

The temperature rise caused in these two situations will *not* be the same, however. A high rate of production, even for a brief time, is likely to cause a greater temperature rise than a lower rate, spread over a longer time. The reason is that more significant cooling can occur during longer, slower exposures. The automatic tube overload prevention devices installed in modern X-ray generators reflect this difference. High value combinations of kV and mA are allowed only for brief exposure times; larger quantities of X-radiation may only be produced more slowly and at a lower rate.

### Rating charts

Before automatic devices became common, radiographers had to consult graphs which displayed the maximum safe kV, mA and exposure time

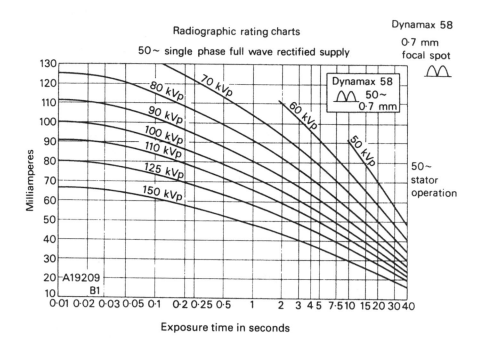

**Fig. 1.17** A typical X-ray tube rating chart. The maximum, safe combinations of kV, mA and exposure time are shown for single exposures. Intersections of mA and time co-ordinates which lie below the kV limiting line are considered *safe* if the anode has not been previously (recently) heated. Note that exposure time is displayed on a logarithmic scale. Charts are valid only for quoted focal spot sizes of the particular type of X-ray tube, operating from a given voltage waveform (the symbol here indicates a 2-pulse supply) at a specified frequency (50 Hz). Note also the unexpectedly limited maximum mA values at 50 kV (below 10 s) and 60 kV (below 2 s): the restrictions are imposed to minimize filament wear when boosted heating is required to offset the space charge effect. (*By courtesy of IGE Medical Systems.*)

combinations. These were known as rating charts. These are now obsolete: they have no role to play in clinical practice, but they may help some students to understand the facts just mentioned.

Rating charts illustrate:

(1)  The reducing availability of higher mA values, as kV is increased;
(2)  The decline of safe mA values available, for a given kV, as exposure times are lengthened;
(3)  A more comparable limitation of available mA values, at longer exposure times, for most kilovoltages, when the rising temperature of the whole anode reduces the temperature gradient between the focal track and its surroundings.

Rating charts may still appear in manufacturers' technical data sheets, in sets for each individual tube, according to:

(1) The type of anode – fixed or rotating;
(2) Speed of disc rotation;
(3) Focal spot size;
(4) Disc design features – composition, size, anode angle;
(5) Nature of the electrical supply to the tube – rectification waveform and frequency.

### Tube power

The rate at which X-rays and heat are produced may otherwise be expressed as the tube's power – the rate of conversion of energy. The maximum safe power will change according to circumstances, chiefly the influence of accumulated heat. For this reason, tube power (*nominal anode input power*) is specified at a standardized exposure time of 0.1 s. In other words, the power expresses the maximum safe rate of X-ray production when the anode is simultaneously having its temperature raised by heat production, at that rate, for a period of 0.1 s.

So, for example, an X-ray tube may be described as having a power of 60 kW or 80 kW (kilowatts). In such cases, it may be expected that the generator which supplies its energy has a comparable power rating.

### The influence of anode temperature

A tube anode can only accept the production of a certain quantity of heat, before its temperature reaches a danger level. Once its temperature starts to rise, cooling begins via the pathways built into the tube's design. Due to the sudden nature of the heat production which occurs during an X-ray exposure, however, it is to be expected that, even with an efficient system, the rate of cooling is lower than the rate of heating. The effect of this imbalance is that the anode's temperature will slowly rise due to the accumulation of heat. If an exposure is made onto an anode which is already at a high temperature, due to residual heat from previous exposures, there is a risk that the safe maximum temperature may be exceeded and that damage will occur.

Older automatic tube overload prevention devices protect the tube, only on the assumption that the anode is cool – that is, not still at a high temperature, following a previous exposure. This assumption may be unjustified.

To inform the radiographer about its current state, heat sensors were incorporated within the tube, transmitting a signal to a display on the generator console or direct to the exposure circuitry. These have been superseded by computer-memory systems which keep a constant check on heating and cooling factors.

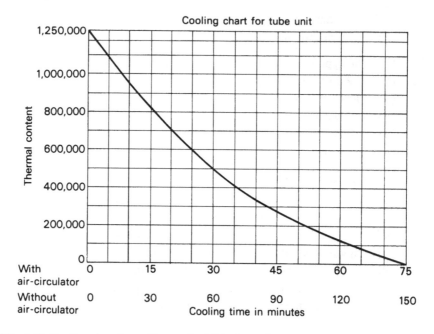

**Fig. 1.18** Cooling chart for an X-ray tube. This shows the rate at which the tube loses heat, with and without fan-assisted air circulation.

### Fluoroscopic rating

When an X-ray tube is used for fluoroscopy – that is, continuous, low intensity exposure, rather than short and intense radiographic exposures – heat accumulation is *gradual*. The resulting temperature rise may spread to the whole tube, rather than just the anode. In other words, the temperature gradient from the target may be very shallow. Confirmation of this may be found in the fact that the anode may either remain motionless or else rotate only at a slow speed.

The pressure-sensitive switch operated by the tube's oil expansion diaphragm or bellows is a safety precaution against tube damage, in these circumstances. Its action is not a fine and immediate response, however, and, again, more accurate devices based on direct temperature monitoring are required in situations where a tube is to be used close to its safety limits.

### *Tube preparation*

Student radiographers soon learn that before a radiographic exposure can be made, the X-ray tube has to be **prepared** ('prepped'). The preparation stage involves a short, compulsory delay, preventing an exposure from being made immediately, even though pressure may be applied to the exposure switch.

### Filament protection

With all X-ray tubes, the preparation period involves heating the filament up to its full operating temperature. Between exposures, the filament is kept at a low, stand-by temperature. It is not kept switched off and cold, so that it can be spared the repeated stress of a full rise and fall, from cold to hot and back again. Neither is the filament kept, between exposures, at its full emission temperature. This temperature would, in any case, vary according to the required tube current, but its relatively high value would also harm the filament, if maintained for long periods of time.

Vaporized loss of tungsten from the filament's surface (not to be confused with thermionic emission of electrons, which are replaced) occurs at a higher rate when its temperature rises. This loss from the surface makes the filament thinner. It thus reduces both the cross-sectional area and the surface area of the wire. Reduction of the surface area lowers the filament's capacity for emitting electrons. Reduction of the cross-sectional area increases electrical resistance, reducing the current which flows through it (for a given potential difference across it), thus further cutting the rate of emission. Uncorrected, the practical outcome of this wear is a reduction in X-ray beam intensity. It is usual for this effect of filament ageing to be offset by corrective compensation in the filament heating circuitry. This involves raising the filament's operating temperatures, however, so that, although emission is sustained, the wearing process is accelerated.

It is important, therefore, that the filament is boosted to its full operating temperature for as short a time as possible before an exposure is made. At the end of an exposure, filament heating is automatically cut back to its stand-by level.

### Anode rotation

With a rotating anode tube, the preparation time is also designed to allow the anode to start moving and accelerate up to its full rotational speed. In this case too, a prolonged preparation time subjects the tube to a risk of unnecessary harm, by increasing wear on the rotation mechanism.

When new, an anode's rotation is smooth and barely audible. With age, it tends to become noisier. Whatever its state, the tube's noise deserves the radiographer's routine attention. If, for some reason, an electrical fault failed to make the anode rotate, an exposure could be made onto a motionless disc, concentrating the whole of the heat on a single area instead of spreading it around the focal track. The temperature rise ensuing from such an accident would probably cause severe damage to the disc.

### Tungsten deposit

Even normal, moderate use of an X-ray tube produces vaporization of tungsten, from both filament and anode. This can contaminate the vacuum and cause a thin film of tungsten to become deposited on the insert's internal parts. In an insert taken from an old tube, this is visible only on the (previously clear) glass wall of the insert, in mild cases, as a pink-brown discoloration. In severe instances, the glass may actually appear silvered.

If this deposit occurs in line with the emission of the useful X-ray beam, between target and window, it may marginally reduce the beam intensity. A more serious problem may arise if the deposit forms a conducting area and becomes electrically charged. In this case, it forms virtually a third electrode and raises the risk of a discharge current which could puncture the envelope, allow entry of oil, and bring the tube's working life to a rapid end.

### Warm-up procedure

The temperature gradient between the focal track and the remainder of the anode disc plays an important part in cooling the focal track. It is possible, however, for this gradient to be the cause of unnecessary stress – in cases where heavy exposures are made on a cold anode. To lessen such stresses and a risk of cracking of the disc, it is common practice to precede a working session with some *warm-up* exposures. The purpose is to produce heat slowly so that the whole disc experiences a small, gradual temperature rise. This procedure is safe, since although X-rays are produced, the tube diaphragms are firmly closed beforehand and no persons are allowed near the tube. Once the tube has been in use, the warm-up requirement is normally fulfilled by residual heat from previous exposures.

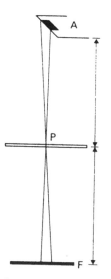

**Fig. 1.19** Principle of the pinhole camera. A pinhole, P, in a sheet of lead equidistant between the tube target, A, and a film, F, can be used to create a true size image of area from which the X-ray beam appears to be produced.

## *Testing*

Tube wear will tend to be accompanied by a progressive reduction in the intensity of its X-ray output. It may also show itself by an enlargement of the focal spot size. Periodic tests may therefore be valuable in monitoring the tube's condition – comparing it with baselines, established when newly purchased and installed.

A simple *pinhole camera* type of test can be carried out to produce an image of the tube's focal spot. This tends not to be very accurate, however, unless very precise equipment is used, both for forming and measuring the image.

Since focal spot dimensions govern the size of penumbra, more suitable and reproducible tests employ controlled production and measurement of penumbra in its visible form: geometric unsharpness of the image of a test object. A wide range of commercial devices can now be purchased to meet this purpose. When used, it is important to recognize that the tube's focal spot size is the effective focal area measured along the central ray. If measured towards the cathode side, it will appear larger, while measured across towards the anode, it will be smaller.

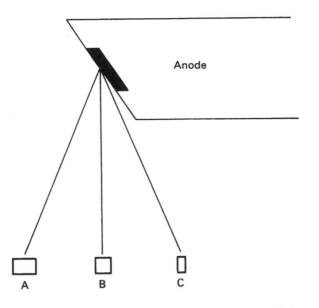

**Fig. 1.20** Perceptions of an X-ray tube's true focal area. B is the tube's effective focal area (*focal spot*). Measured at A, the X-ray source appears larger. At C, it is smaller.

## 1.7 Follow-up practical

(1) Examine closely any parts of dismantled X-ray tubes. There are usually several, somewhere in a clinical department – possibly in a separate education room or museum. Only by handling tube components, can their size, shape and relationships become apparent.

(2) Take a good look at all the X-ray tubes which are in use in your clinical department. Differences between them – for instance, some will be larger than others – are likely to be due to the different purposes which they serve, and may be matched by the various, different generators which power them.

(3) Follow up your observations by looking at the manufacturers' leaflets and technical material supplied with the tubes. From these documents you will be able to discover a tube's exact specifications: its focal spot sizes, rate of anode rotation, anode disc composition, power, etc. Try to learn why particular tubes have been installed in the various rooms; are the reasons linked to the techniques practised in those rooms; or because of the other equipment with which it operates?

(4) At a generator control panel which is not too automated, investigate the various combinations of tube kilovoltage, milliamperage and exposure time which (a) can be used safely or (b) are not allowed. What does this information tell you about the X-ray tube?

(5) Familiarize yourself with the methods in use in the department, to warm up tubes before a working session; and to test tubes, as part of the quality assurance programme.

(6) How are test results (not only for tubes but for *all* the equipment described in this book) recorded? Each room or unit should have its own record book for charting the equipment's performance and maintenance – showing, by implication, its reliability, safety and cost-effectiveness.

# Part Two
# X-Ray Generators

Unlike most domestic electrical appliances, X-ray tubes cannot simply be plugged into the mains voltage supply. An X-ray tube requires two or three different supplies which must also be adjustable, to control the X-ray output, suiting it to its various clinical purposes. An X-ray tube, therefore, recieves its electrical supplies from an X-ray **generator**.

From observation and use of the various facilities on its control panel, students will already be familiar with the outward appearance of an X-ray generator. The inner workings of the generator will be less familiar. They may, indeed, represent an awesome challenge, especially to those with limited previous experience of studying electrical science. To assist such students in particular, the three chapters which together form this part of the text have been centred on the three principal generator control variables (*exposure factors*): tube kilovoltage, tube current and exposure time.

# Chapter 2
# Control of the X-Ray Tube Kilovoltage

## 2.1 Introduction

From studying the X-ray tube, students will already know that an electrical potential difference of several thousands of volts is required to make the tube work. The production of this potential difference – the tube kilovoltage (kV) – is probably the most significant function of an X-ray generator. It is certainly the commonest feature by which any X-ray generator is identified.

Methods of kilovoltage production have changed considerably, over the years. Although the change has been gradual, some methods of generating tube kilovoltage are now virtually obsolete; their shortcomings can serve a purpose, however: to confirm the superiority of the modern generator.

### The need for a kilovoltage

X-rays are produced as a result of energy conversion: from the kinetic energy possessed by electrons crossing the X-ray tube, into X-rays. This kinetic energy is itself a conversion product – from the potential energy which the electrons possess while still in the vicinity of the filament.

The kilovoltage applied across the X-ray tube gives these electrons their potential energy. As they begin to move across to the tube's anode, it becomes their kinetic energy. In order to produce X-rays, the electrons' kinetic energy must be considerable. Its threshold value – below which X-rays cannot be produced, but above which, they can – is difficult to identify. For clinical purposes, this is largely academic, since all of the kilovoltage values offered by a generator will cause the X-ray tube to produce X-rays. As a general guide, this range will usually lie between 40 kV and 130 kV.

### The need for kilovoltage variation

Students will know that an X-ray generator offers its user a range of kilovoltage values. Why should kilovoltage variation be necessary? There are two principal reasons. Both arise from the kilovoltage's role as provider of the X-ray beam's energy.

**(1)** When they interact with the X-ray tube target, electrons from the filament may have their kinetic energy converted into photons of X-rays. Production of a photon causes an electron to lose some of its kinetic energy. The possession of more kinetic energy (due to a higher tube kilovoltage) can enable electrons to produce photons of greater X-ray energy. Compared with less energetic photons, these are capable of greater penetration: they can pass through structures which are more radiopaque.

Thus, a simple answer lies in the need for X-ray penetration. A survey of the kilovoltage values used for radiography of a range of anatomical subjects – from a finger to an abdomen – reveals an obvious link: the more opaque the structure, the higher the selected kilovoltage. The term more usually employed to define an X-ray beam's penetrating ability, is its **quality**. This may be interpreted as indicating the most commonly occurring photon energy within an X-ray beam; if this value is raised – for example, by kilovoltage selection – the beam's quality is higher.

**(2)** The greater kinetic energy acquired by electrons crossing the X-ray tube at higher values of kilovoltage may also result in the production of more X-ray photons. Each electron may, at its greater speed, be able to interact with more tube target atoms before losing its given energy. Because of their higher average energy, more photons are able to pass through the tube's inherent filtration, to join the beam which emerges from the tube window. The presence of more photons in an X-ray beam, at any given time, raises the property of an X-ray beam known as its **intensity**. This is defined as the rate of flow of X-ray energy through a unit area lying at 90° to the path of the beam.

By use of a higher tube kilovoltage to increase the energy of the electron beam flowing through the tube, the rate of flow of X-ray energy out of the tube – that is, the beam's intensity – is increased. This facility may be used by a radiographer in order to achieve a reduction in the time required for an exposure, and so reduce the chance of image blur due to movement.

There are other benefits from having a range of kilovoltages to choose from. These concern control of image contrast and radiation protection. More relevant to this present discussion, however, is the matter of how choice of a given kilovoltage value is achieved.

## 2.2 Voltage transformation

Mains voltage is insufficient for X-ray production: if applied across the X-ray tube, it would fail to give filament electrons the required kinetic energy for conversion into X-rays. An increase up to the required kilovoltage is achieved quite easily, however, by the use of a common and familiar electrical device: a **transformer**.

A conventional transformer has three principal components:

(1) A primary winding: the coiled length of wire across which the primary voltage (the value which is to be changed) is applied.
(2) A secondary winding: the coiled length of wire across which the secondary voltage (the required, eventual value) is induced.
(3) A central magnetic core, around which both windings are arranged.

The voltage relationship between primary and secondary is established by the phenomenon of electromagnetic induction. The current flowing through the primary winding, in response to the applied primary voltage, sets up a magnetic field. Because the voltage is alternating, the current alternates and its magnetic field varies in its polarity (north/south/north, etc.) at the same rate.

Faraday's laws of electromagnetic induction predict the outcome within the secondary winding. Under the influence of the changing magnetic field (conserved and enhanced by the transformer's core), an electromotive force – a voltage or kilovoltage – is induced across the secondary winding.

The ratio between the applied, primary voltage and the induced secondary voltage is determined by the transformer's **turns ratio**, between the number of turns (around the core) forming the respective primary and secondary windings.

It is important to realize that there is *no* electrical *conducting* link between the primary and secondary windings: the electron flow around each winding is intact; it has no connection with the other.

A transformer which converts a relatively low voltage into a higher value is said to *step up* the voltage. Conversely, a voltage reduction is achieved by a *step down* transformer.

### *The high tension transformer*

The transformer used for generating a kilovoltage across the X-ray tube is fed by a relatively low voltage which it increases or *steps up*. Due to the magnitude of its output, this particular transformer is usually known as the generator's *high tension* (HT) transformer. *Tension* is an old-fashioned term for potential difference. Its use has tended to become obsolete except with reference to this transformer and its secondary circuit.

The electrical risks associated with the kilovoltages required for X-ray production make it essential for the HT transformer to be very fully insulated and, as with the X-ray tube, mounted within a shockproofed housing. In common with an X-ray tube, an HT transformer becomes hot during use. It is therefore usually also immersed in oil which serves as both an insulator and convectant. The HT transformer is housed together with the tube filament transformer (also at high tension, through its connection to the cathode) within the generator's transformer *tank*.

It could be possible for the X-ray tube to be supplied simply by a kilovoltage resulting from a stepped up mains voltage. This simplicity would ignore two important facts, however:

(1) Supplied direct from the mains, the HT transformer's output – in other words, the kilovoltage across the X-ray tube – would be fixed, denying the radiographer an opportunity to vary its value. (Moreover, any temporary fluctuations occurring in the mains voltage would be passed on by the transformer, so that kilovoltage variation, if and when it occurred, would be beyond the radiographer's control.)

(2) Because the voltage output from the transformer is (necessarily) alternating, the polarity across the X-ray tube would also alternate: the anode, which must be at positive potential to attract the filament electrons, would actually be negative, half the time. Equally, during alternate intervals, the cathode would be positive.

The need to achieve a controllable kilovoltage and eliminate the effect of mains fluctuations is met by having a carefully designed circuit to supply the HT transformer's primary winding.

## 2.3 The high tension primary circuit

### The autotransformer

When considering a conventional transformer, it may be overlooked that the changing magnetic field created by the primary current also induces an electromotive force (emf) in the primary winding itself. This fact is crucial to the basic design of the autotransformer: it only has *one* winding around its core.

A second peculiar feature concerns access to, that is, the facility for making connections to, this single winding. Conventionally, connections can only be made to the ends of a transformer's windings. If the transformer is employed to change a supply voltage by a fixed factor, there is no purpose in having any other connection points. In contrast to this, an auto-transformer's single winding is interrupted *along its length* by connection access points, known as **tappings**. By the use of these, both its input connections (from the mains) and output connections (to the HT transformer) can be varied. In other words, its turns ratio is *widely variable*. This allows it to provide the required facilities of mains voltage compensation and kilovoltage selection.

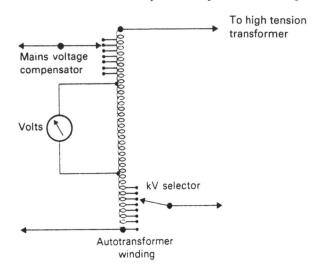

**Fig. 2.1** The autotransformer. The autotransformer has sets of tappings both on its *primary* side, for variable connection of input mains voltage (to compensate for fluctuations) and its *secondary* side, for variation of its output supply to the high tension transformer (to generate required values of kilovoltage).

### Mains voltage compensation

Mains voltage supplies are quoted as **nominal** values. When circumstances are ideal, the actual value of the voltage is this nominal figure (in the UK, 240 or 415 V, root mean square, depending on the connection to the supply lines). When electricity demands are high, however, and when they suddenly change, the electricity supply stations cannot always maintain this nominal value. The actual value may then drop below or rise above the nominal value. This unwelcome, up-or-down variation is known as **fluctuation**.

Domestic consumers are rarely aware of mains voltage fluctuations. Most household electrical appliances are unlikely to be affected in their functions. This is not true of X-ray equipment. Fluctuations can cause the quality and intensity of the X-ray beam to be affected, with consequent effects on diagnostic radiographic images.

Mains voltage is applied across the autotransformer, from one chosen point or tapping to another. Its effect is to produce a current through the turns of the autotransformer which lie between these two points. The current establishes a changing magnetic field which induces an emf across the whole of the autotransformer. This whole emf may be considered to be the sum of the separate, equal values induced across each turn. Whatever this volts-per-turn value is (say, 2 V), it is important that it should remain accurate and constant so that the autotransformer can act as a reliable voltage source for the various circuits within the generator.

This reliability is threatened by mains fluctuations. A rise in mains voltage will increase the current flowing through the turns which lie between the points of application. Its magnetic effect will be stronger and the induced emf will increase proportionately. In other words, the mains voltage fluctuation will pass through to the generator.

This problem is overcome by a variation of the length of the auto-transformer winding – the number of turns – across which the mains voltage is connected. If this length is varied in proportion to the actual, instantaneous value of the mains voltage, there will be a consistency in the current through the autotransformer, the induced emf per turn, and the performance of the generator.

Mains voltage is thus applied across the autotransformer via variable tappings which change in harmony with fluctuations, as they occur. The control over these variable tappings, the mains voltage compensator, operates in conjunction with a detector which monitors and feeds back information to the compensator about the mains voltage – whether it is at, below or above its nominal value.

Older generators were equipped with manually operated mains voltage compensators. In these, the link between the monitoring device and the compensator was provided by the radiographer's observation. Usually, a simple meter displayed the state of the mains voltage; the radiographer responded to the display by using the manually-operated control to adjust the transformer connection to a different tapping, if necessary.

The potential weakness of this arrangement was, of course, that the radiographer's attention could have been focused elsewhere – typically and understandably on the patient – so that occasionally an exposure was made without adequate compensation. The outcome may have been incorrect image quality.

A modern generator has fully automatic circuitry which removes the possibility of this human error. A voltage-sensitive device continuously monitors the mains supply. Its readings are fed to a motor-driven compensator which instantly responds, connecting the mains voltage, at its new value, across more or fewer turns of the autotransformer, exactly as required. Because it is an automatic function, there is no evidence on the generator console about its presence. The student should be aware of its existence, however, if only through being reassured that mains voltage fluctuations cannot disturb image quality.

## Kilovoltage selection

The fixed nature of the HT transformer's turns ratio has already been described. Whatever the value of the input voltage, the output is a stepped up, fixed multiple. There is no facility for varying the factor by which the primary is transformed in to the secondary. This fixed relationship is inescapable, due to the magnitude of the transformer's output: the high tension, or kilovoltage. Insulation of electrical conductors is required in proportion to the potential difference which is applied between the conductors and their surroundings – whether these are other conductors or persons who wish to remain safe from an electric shock. It would hardly be possible for tappings to be provided on the HT transformer, to vary its turns ratio; the insulation precautions required would make such an arrangement very awkward both to construct and operate. Instead, the output from the HT transformer, the kilovoltage, is varied simply by adjusting the value of the input voltage, from the autotransformer. A control which incorporates a range of tappings is provided on the autotransformer to allow the voltage from more or fewer turns to be selected. Although this control actually deals only with relatively low voltages, their automatic transformation into kilovoltages explains why it is known as the kilovoltage selector.

The provision of a kilovoltage selector alone is not enough for the radiographer; there has to be some indication of the selected value. The manner in which kilovoltage is indicated differs from one control panel to another. Most commonly, this display is digital, possibly on a combined visual display screen.

Actual measurement of the selected kilovoltage may, as with its selection, be achieved within the low voltage section of the generator which provides the primary supply to the HT transformer. This arrangement is electrically simple and safe: the measuring device is connected across the voltage supplied to the HT transformer primary winding. Being at low voltage (rather than in the secondary circuit, with all its potential hazards) it can be on the generator's control panel. Display of kilovoltage is possible through employing the principle of calibration.

Calibrated display devices are found in many situations. The speedometer on a motor vehicle's dashboard, for example, is actually measuring the small electrical current produced by the rotation of the vehicle's road wheels. This actual information would be of no value to the driver – no more than knowledge of the actual voltage being fed to the HT transformer would be to a radiographer. Instead, in the case of a vehicle, an interpretation of the current values into the speeds which generate them is built into the meter. It is said to be **calibrated**.

In the X-ray generator, the low voltage is actually displayed in a calibrated form, as the kilovoltage which it will surely become when it has been transformed.

## 2.4 The need for rectification

Generation of a kilovoltage is not, by itself, a complete answer to the need for a high potential difference across the X-ray tube. The mains voltage is an alternating supply – in fact, a transformer cannot operate unless its supply is alternating – and the kilovoltage output from the HT transformer is also alternating.

To operate efficiently, an X-ray tube should be fed with a kilovoltage which has a fixed polarity, so that its anode is consistently at a high positive potential, and its cathode is negative. Even so, it is possible for an X-ray tube to operate even if its supply is alternating. A brief, progressive review of this and other inadequate arrangements will helpfully underline the near-ideal features of a modern generator.

## *Self-rectification*

The most noticeable drawback to operating an X-ray tube from an alternating voltage supply is the fact that during alternate half-cycles, when the anode is negative and the cathode positive, there is no tube current. Electrons from the filament will not be attracted across the tube while the anode has a negative potential; and the anode, not being equipped with a filament, cannot produce electrons to flow across to a positive cathode. During these alternate half-cycles, therefore, there is no X-ray production.

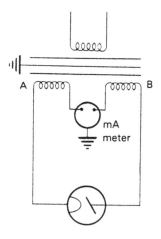

Fig. 2.2 Self-rectification. The output kilovoltage alternating its polarity across the high tension transformer's secondary winding, AB, is applied across the X-ray tube without intermediate rectification.

By allowing current to flow through it in one direction only, despite having an alternating potential difference applied across it, the X-ray tube is acting as a rectifier. Because this action prevents a reverse current without external aid, the tube is said to be operating under **self-rectification** conditions.

The self-rectifying action of an X-ray tube can be rather precarious, however. While it is true that the anode is not designed to be an emitter of electrons, bombardment of the target by electrons to produce X-rays also generates heat. Thus, after it has been in use for even a short period, the anode's temperature rises and introduces the risk that electron emission will occur. If a reversed potential difference is then applied (anode negative, cathode positive) a reverse current will flow; the rectifying action will be lost. The effect of electron bombardment on the cathode will be a rise in temperature – which the cathode is not designed to tolerate. There is also a risk of X-ray production, but the the likelihood of permanent damage and loss of function is more significant.

Despite these drawbacks, self-rectification was, at one time, a popular and workable proposition: it offered a cheap and compact arrangement for low powered production of X-rays. (Power being the rate of conversion of energy from one form to another, a low rate of X-ray production was accompanied by a low rate of heat production.) Self-rectified equipment may still be used, even today, for dental radiography. The low power does not justify the use of a rotating anode tube. A fixed anode tube is used, therefore, enclosed together with its supply transformers in a **single tank housing**.

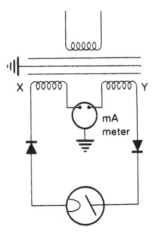

**Fig. 2.3** Half-wave rectification. Two rectifiers in series with the X-ray tube suppress inverse half-cycles of the high tension transformer output voltage, when X is at positive potential and Y is at negative potential.

## *Half-wave rectification*

The task of rectification – of allowing current to flow in one direction only, despite the application of an alternating potential difference – is performed in all other X-ray generators by purpose-built rectifiers, not by the tube itself.

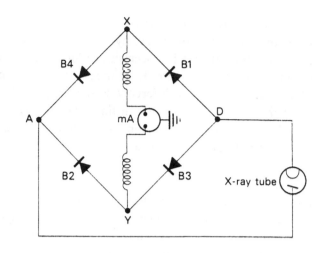

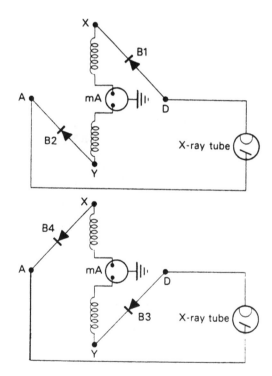

(a)

(b)

**Fig. 2.4** Full-wave (two-pulse) rectification. (a) The HT transformer output across XY is routed by rectifiers B1, 2, 3 and 4, to produce a constant polarity across AD and thus across the X-ray tube. (b) The rectifiers operate in pairs, to conduct alternate half-cycles: B1 and B2, when X is negative and Y is positive; B3 and B4, when Y is negative and X is positive.

The simplest of these generators involves the connection of two rectifiers in series with the tube. The inverse voltage is thus applied not across the tube alone, but across tube plus rectifiers. By preventing a reverse current, this overcomes the risk of damage to the cathode; the anode temperature can rise safely above the point at which thermionic emission occurs, but not so high as to cause thermal damage to the target.

This arrangement does not solve the problem of alternate, non-conducting half-cycles; X-ray production is still intermittent.

### Full-wave rectification: the two-pulse generator

The use of four rectifiers, arranged as a *bridge*, is the classic method of manoeuvring an alternating potential difference so that it is applied across any given device – in this case, an X-ray tube – with a constant polarity. Thus the situation in which the anode is positive and the cathode negative is achieved consistently, during every half cycle. The sine-wave supply is fully rectified and (hence the generator's name) there are two pulses of X-rays per cycle.

## 2.5 Shortcomings of a pulsating X-ray supply

In the generator circuit just described, the duration of a kilovoltage pulse is half a cycle – in the UK, 0.01 s. Close consideration of the situation will reveal, however, that the pulse of X-rays is shorter than this. From the start of a half-cycle, kilovoltage climbs from zero, towards its peak value. Production of X-rays does not begin, however, until the kilovoltage reaches an arbitrary value – say, 40 or 45 – and ceases when the kilovoltage falls below this value, as it again approaches zero. Even above this threshold, depending on the anatomical structure being radiographed, X-rays may be produced which are incapable of penetrating through to the image formation plane.

The pulse of useful, image-forming X-rays may therefore be considerably shorter than 0.01 s. In other words, although rectification has produced a continuous kilovoltage polarity, X-ray production is still intermittent. Worse than this, during the intervals between zero and the start/finish of a useful pulse, X-rays are being produced which have low energy, destined only to be absorbed by the patient and increase the biological hazard. Below the threshold kilovoltage value for X-ray production, the only energy conversion which occurs at the target is from the electrons' kinetic energy, into heat – unprofitably raising or maintaining its temperature.

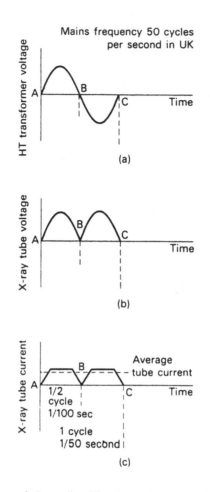

**Fig. 2.5** Full-wave (two-pulse) supplies. The alternating output from the HT transformer (a) is rectified (b) before being applied across the X-ray tube. Intermittency of tube current (c) due to pulsation of the potential difference across the tube results in a correspondingly intermittent X-ray output. Each radiation pulse occupies a period shorter than the duration of a half-cycle. Due to its fluctuation, the tube current has an average (mean) below its maximum (saturation) value.

## The use of capacitors

The voltage waveform may be **smoothed** – that is, have its range limited, to the upper values – by connecting capacitors in parallel with the X-ray tube. This arrangement raises the average kilovoltage across the tube and helps to eliminate the undesirable effects associated with lower values.

Another use of capacitors is to charge them up to the required peak kilovoltage and then use their discharge through the tube, to produce X-rays. This type of generator may be found useful for mobile X-ray units. It has the considerable advantage of consistency: every exposure made at a

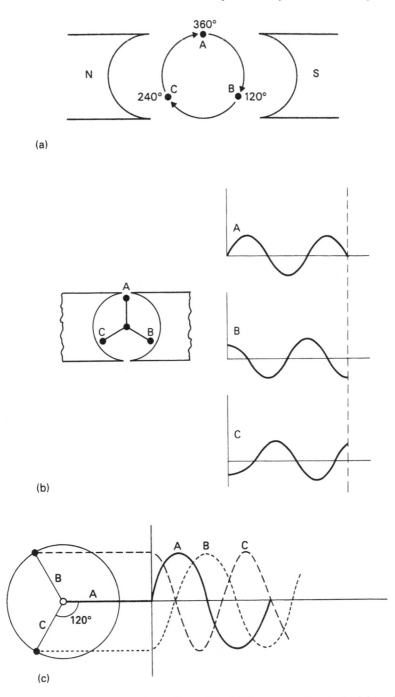

**Fig. 2.6** Generation of three voltage phases. The 120° separation (spacing) of the coils within a voltage generator (a) results in an output of three independent sine waves (b) which are 120° out of phase with each other. This phase difference may equally well be expressed as a time separation: one-third of a cycle. Superimposed on a single graph (c) the continuity of supply offered by these three phases is clear.

given kilovoltage setting is identical, unaffected by mains voltage variations. The only influence which mains variation can have, is on the charging phase, not on the discharging.

## Three-phase generators

### The three-phase supply system

The problem of filling the intervals between the X-ray pulses from a two-pulse generator was solved when an X-ray generator was invented which employed the whole of the mains electricity supply, not just one or two of its phases.

The full output from an electricity supply service comprises three identical, sine-wave supplies. The three phases do not rise and fall simultaneously: they are out of phase with each other by an interval of a third of a cycle. This difference is normally expressed with reference to the rotary principle of voltage generation: one-third of a rotation, i.e. 120°.

When rectified, in a manner similar to the two-pulse generator, each phase supplies two pulses per cycle, giving a total of six per cycle – a six-pulse generator.

By use of two high tension transformer secondary windings (differently wound) instead of just one, the output applied across the tube can be doubled up to 12 pulses per cycle. This kilovoltage waveform, instead of pulsating, is described as rippling. It clearly solves the problem of unpro-

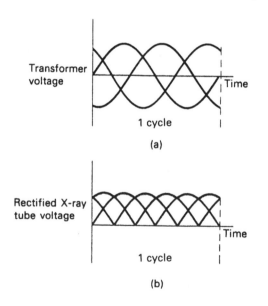

Fig. 2.7 Three-phase voltage rectification. Alternate half-cycles of each waveform are inverted, to produce six *forward* or positive voltage pulses per cycle.

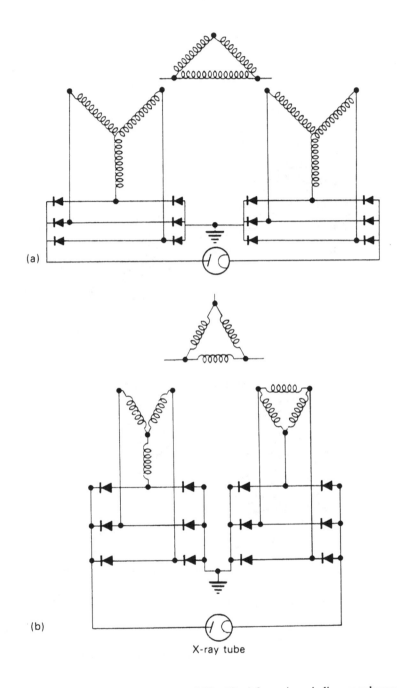

**Fig. 2.8** Three-phase rectification. *Delta* and *Wye* (*Star*) formation windings may be used to generate in-phase (a) or out-of-phase (b) effects, to reduce the magnitude of voltage ripple across the X-ray tube.

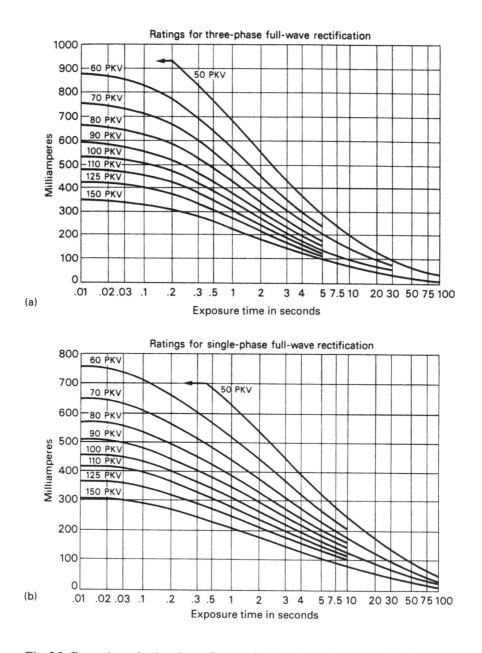

(a)

(b)

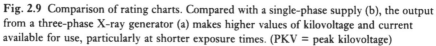

**Fig. 2.9** Comparison of rating charts. Compared with a single-phase supply (b), the output from a three-phase X-ray generator (a) makes higher values of kilovoltage and current available for use, particularly at shorter exposure times. (PKV = peak kilovoltage)

ductive intervals, giving an almost continuous supply of kilovoltage at its selected peak value.

It should be noted that the use of a three-phase supply, while achieving an almost constant potential across the tube, still results in an X-ray beam which contains low energy photons. The random bremsstrahlung profile, the continuous spectrum, is still produced – although, compared with single-phase operation, it contains a greater proportion of higher energy photons. In other words, the beam quality is higher. Due also to the higher average photon energy, the beam intensity is greater than from a single-phase generator, using identical mA and kV settings.

Compared with a single-phase generator, a difference can be seen in the tube rating permitted by a three-phase kilovoltage supply – that is, the maximum safe combinations of mA, kV and exposure time. The greater efficiency of the electrical supply to the tube raises the average values, bringing them nearer to the limiting peak values.

## High frequency generators

The modern, standard solution to the challenge of producing an unbroken beam of X-rays is based on conversion of the standard mains voltage frequency, e.g. from 50 Hz (UK) up to values in the thousands (i.e. thousands of cycles per second). This type of generator produces high output and accuracy, while being considerably smaller than an older, low frequency generator.

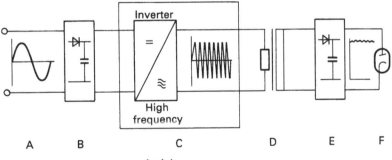

High-frequency generator principle

Fig. 2.10 Principle of the high frequency X-ray generator. The input voltage (A) is rectified and smoothed with capacitors (B). It is then fed to a circuit which reconverts it to an alternating voltage by the action of an inverter, but now at a high frequency (C). This high frequency voltage is transformed up to the required kilovoltage (D), rectified and smoothed (E) for application across the X-ray tube (F). (*By courtesy of Siemens plc.*)

The key to reduction in size lies in the conversion to high frequency. Faraday's second law of electromagnetic induction states that the magnitude of the induced electromotive force is directly proportional to the rate of change of magnetic flux. Conversion of the primary voltage to a high frequency supply before it is fed to the HT transformer enables it to generate kilovoltages with greatly increased efficiency. The practical consequence of this is that, for an output equivalent to a conventional, low frequency transformer, the high frequency transformer is very much smaller. The reduction in size may be so marked that the transformer may be included with the X-ray tube insert, in a single tank.

## 2.6 High tension cables

The kilovoltage generated by the high tension transformer and subsequently rectified has to be transmitted for application across the X-ray tube. If transformer and tube are together within a single tank, the task is simple: only short connectors, properly insulated, are required.

If the X-ray tube is remote from the generator, the task is greater: this distance must be bridged by cables, flexible to permit movement of the tube but also free from the risk of electrical hazards. Students will already be familiar with the external appearance of HT cables. The internal design is determined by the purposes the cables must serve:

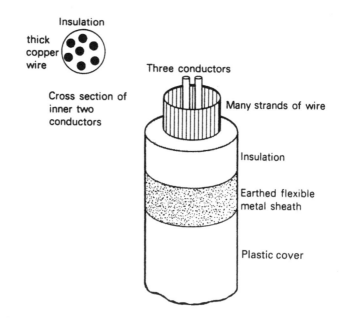

Fig. 2.11 High tension cable. The three central conductors are shown as two inner, closely grouped wires, with an outer, circular third conductor.

(1) The tube current must be conducted between tube and rectifiers with a minimal drop in its value. The conductors with the HT cables must therefore have an appropriately low resistance. Since the tube current rarely exceeds 1 A and filament currents typically range from 3 A–6 A, this requirement is easily met by relatively normal copper wires.

(2) Another supply, also at high tension, has to be fed to the X-ray tube. This is the voltage from the tube filament transformers to the tube filaments. Two conductors per filament are required for the circulation of the filament current. For the standard, dual-focus X-ray tube, this requirement would seem to imply that four conductors are required. In fact, three conductors suffice: one each for the two filaments, and one *common* – used, in turn, by either. This common conductor is also used for conduction of the tube current.

(3) All conductors need to be insulated. The potential difference across a tube filament is typically about 20 V. The filament supply conductors therefore need only fairly thin mutual insulation. But these conductors, because of their connection to the strongly negative cathode, are at a considerable potential difference with respect to earth – up to 75 kV. **Earth** or **ground** is the zero electrical potential of the patient, members of staff and all the outer, metallic parts of the equipment. It is clear, therefore, that a considerable thickness of insulation is required around all the conductors within an HT cable. The insulation stress is cut to half the potential difference across the X-ray tube, by the midpoint earthing of the HT transformer's secondary winding. Even so, it remains high enough to require a thickness of insulating material which is much greater than is ever required in the flex supplying a domestic electrical appliance.

(4) For the electrical safety of an HT cable, reliance on insulation alone would contravene safety requirements. Plastic and rubber can be accidentally cut or abraded and, with age, can become friable. As a guarantee of safety, therefore, HT cables are shockproofed. Their insulation is surrounded by a metallic sheath at earth potential. If the inner insulation fails, charge from the conductors can then travel to earth via this sheath and not via a person touching the cable or standing nearby.

The cables thus complete the shockproofing which surrounds all equipment components at high tension: transformer and rectifiers, cables and X-ray tube are continuously protected.

(5) Bearing in mind the flexibility and free movement which the cable should have, the insulating layers are kept at a minimal thickness for their purpose; and the shockproofing metallic sheath takes the form of a woven braid or net, rather than being a more solid, rigid layer.

**(6)** In order to be cleanable and hygienic, and smooth when handled, the outermost layer of an HT cable is a continuous sheath of rubber or plastic which also protects the shockproofing layer against damage.

### High tension connections to the tube and generator

At its terminal points, where it is connected to the tube and transformer tank, the flexible insulation in an HT cable is replaced by rigid, mineral or ceramic insulation. Within this, the cable conductors become continuous with rigid metallic rods. These protrude from the cable, to engage with corresponding sockets in the tube and tank ports. Continuity of shock-proofing is achieved by a metallic ring onto which the braiding is soldered. Surrounding it is a threaded collar screwed tightly onto the cable ports at both ends of the cable.

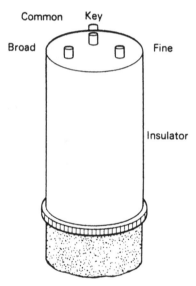

**Fig. 2.12** High tension cable terminal. This fits into an identically reciprocal socket at both the X-ray tube and the high tension transformer tank.

The symmetry of the connecting pins is prevented from allowing misconnection by the use of a **key**. This is a raised ridge along the cable's terminal which must be aligned with a corresponding groove along the receptacle into which it fits.

The special need at the cathode, for separate connections to the filaments, is met by the three central conductors within the cable. Connection to the anode requires only a single conductor. Despite this simplicity, the same type of cable is used for the anode connection as for the cathode. Only one of the inner conductors needs to be used.

## 2.7 Kilovoltage compensation

During an exposure, a high current is drawn from the mains. This may be as high as 100 A, or more. The effect of charge travelling at such a rate along the conductors which bring the mains supply to the X-ray generator is that a voltage drop occurs. A further drop in voltage, proportional to the current, occurs within the HT transformer, due to its regulation. The actual voltage dropped is determined by two factors: the resistance (impedance) of the conductors and the current flowing along them.

The current is largely determined by the value of the tube current in use. If the selected tube current is changed, say, from 400 mA to 700 mA, a proportionately higher current will be drawn from the mains during the exposure, and a proportionately higher voltage drop will occur.

If no compensation is made, this voltage drop will be passed on to the generator, suppressing its functions. Of concern in this context is the effect on the kilovoltage. Without compensation, as the selected tube current is increased or reduced, there would be a reciprocal rise or fall of the kilovoltage, above or below its expected value.

The voltage drop occurring when a given current is drawn from the mains can be calculated beforehand, if the mains resistance (impedance) is known. Compensation can thus be planned and implemented. (It is for this purpose that some mobile X-ray generators incorporate a means of measuring the mains resistance at the various sockets to which it is connected.)

One compensation arrangement is semi-automatic, relying on action by

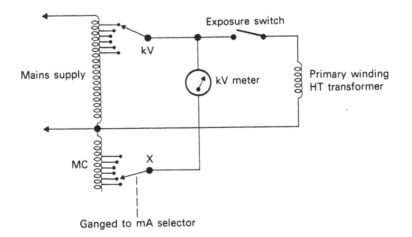

Fig. 2.13 Kilovoltage compensation. Tube current selection may cause a change in the displayed kilovoltage, indicating a need for altering the voltage tapped from the autotransformer via the kV selector.

the radiographer. This is put into action when the displayed value of the selected kV is altered by a change in the selected mA value. Observing this change, the radiographer resets the kV, and the exposure can then be correctly made. The kV meter change is due to a link between the mA selector and the kV meter. This change – a kV drop if the mA is increased; a kV rise if the mA is reduced – predicts the voltage drop effect on kV if no compensation is made. The radiographer's action is to readjust the voltage applied to the HT transformer primary winding, to ensure that the required kV is actually achieved.

More usual, is a fully automatic arrangement, with a compensatory circuit link between the mA selector and the tappings from the autotransformer.

The effect of this compensation is to make the tube kilovoltage independent of the tube current.

### *Testing for correct compensation*

A simple test can be carried out to check the accuracy of the compensation provided by an X-ray generator. The test simply requires a set of exposures of an aluminium step-wedge.

Suitable exposure factors (kilovoltage, milliampere seconds and focus–film distance) are determined which produce an image of the wedge with all its steps clearly visible. Let us suppose that this exposure is 75 kV and 60 mAs.

Several exposures are then made of the step wedge, side by side, across the film, with adjacent unexposed areas protected by collimation and lead masking. The kV and the mAs (product of mA × s) must be the same for each exposure but derive from different mA values and (reciprocally adjusted) exposure times. For example:

| mA × s | mA × s |
|---|---|
| 600 × 0.1 | 300 × 0.2 |
| 500 × 0.12 | 200 × 0.3 |
| 400 × 0.15 | 100 × 0.6 |

Students will notice that the mathematics of this experiment is considerably simplified if an easily factorized number such as 60 is selected. With appropriate adjustment of the focus–film distance (to increase or reduce beam intensity), this should be achievable.

The resultant line of images should show consistent densities, step by step, across from the first exposure to the last. If not, there is a compensation defect and the equipment manufacturer's engineers should be called in, to correct it.

## 2.8 Measuring kilovoltage

An absolute measure of the accuracy of selected kilovoltages lies beyond the daily scope of a radiographer's duties: the high tension cables need to be disconnected from the X-ray tube and applied, instead, to a shockproofed device which will give a direct reading.

Instead, the practical tests available for occasional quality assurance checks actually test the principal beam parameter or property which is controlled by the tube kilovoltage: its quality – specifically, its ability to penetrate a test object.

Also influenced by kilovoltage is the beam's intensity – and test images need to take this into account. Tests are most readily performed to measure kilovoltage on a relative rather than an absolute basis: each repeated test compares tube output with its performance at the previous test. Ideally, the series should date back to the tests carried out when the tube and generator were originally installed.

## 2.9 Follow-up practical

**(1)** Carry out your own survey of the X-ray generators available in your clinical department(s).

(a) What range of kilovoltages are available?
(b) Are the ranges on all the control panels the same?
(c) How are the selected kV values indicated? On scales, screens, meters or by some other means?
(d) Is is clear what type of rectification is produced by the generator?
(e) Familiarize yourself with the use of manually-controlled mains voltage compensation (if available).

**(2)** Investigate the kV values which are used for radiography of various anatomical areas. Is there an obvious proportionality between the kilovoltage and the opacity of the area?

**(3)** Using X-ray (tissue equivalent) phantoms, produce some experimental images, using identical values of kV, mAs, focus–film distance, etc., but using different types of generator.

**(4)** Carry out the test for checking kilovoltage compensation.

**(5)** Using the test equipment available in the clinical department, carry out a measurement of kilovoltage, in accordance with the departmental protocol.

# Chapter 3
# Control of the X-Ray Tube Current

## 3.1 Introduction

X-rays are produced as a result of electrons flowing through an X-ray tube, from a heated filament within the cathode, across to the anode. The rate at which they flow is the X-ray tube current, measured in milliamperes and commonly referred to as simply **the mA**. Tube current directly affects the rate at which X-ray photons are produced and, consequently, the X-ray beam's intensity. The primary reason for needing to have control over tube current, therefore, is to be able to adjust X-ray beam intensity: high tube current giving high beam intensity, lower current giving a reduced intensity.

For most radiographic purposes, an X-ray beam of high intensity is commonly considered to be ideal. It allows exposure times to be minimal and thus reduces the risk of image unsharpness which accompanies any movement the object makes during an exposure.

Produced simultaneously with X-rays, however, is heat. When an intense X-ray beam is produced, therefore, heat production also takes place at a proportionately high rate. In this situation, there is an increased risk of thermal damage to the X-ray tube, particularly to its target or focal track. In practice, therefore, tube current is preset to an appropriate value, high or low, before an exposure is made, in order both to control X-ray beam intensity and protect the X-ray tube against thermal damage.

## 3.2 The need for accuracy

For radiographic purposes, accuracy of tube current – that is, how precisely it meets the preset requirement – is vital. A radiographic exposure may be considered to be an essentially *blind* process since confirmation of its accuracy is delayed until the radiographic image has been processed. This is true whether mA selection is manual – when the radiographer positively selects a certain mA value; or automatic – when mA selection is under electronic control.

Quantities of X-radiation required for creating radiographic images are preselected by use of the peculiarly radiographic unit, the milliampere second (symbol mAs). In fact, this is a unit of electric charge, a milli-coulomb, but its alternative name identifies its dependent factors: tube current (mA) and exposure time, measured in seconds (s). Modern X-ray generators incorporate exposure timers which are accurate to a millisecond. This accuracy must be complemented by accuracy of mA values. Otherwise, quantities of radiation will vary from expected values and frustrate attempts to control both image quality and radiation safety.

## 3.3 Tube filament circuitry

In principle, control of tube current is simple: the filament temperature is raised or lowered to produce the required current, high or low. The simplicity of this arrangement needs to be questioned by the student radiographer, however, for it involves some conditions which must be understood if operation of the X-ray generator is to be informed rather than routine.

### *Passage of the tube current through a vacuum*

An X-ray tube operates when a stream of electrons is conducted through it, across the vacuum, from filament to anode. This phenomenon is sufficiently different from the more usual flow of electrons through a solid conductor (a copper wire, for instance) to deserve a student's attention.

Ohm's law concerning an electric current may be familiar: the application of a potential difference across a solid conductor will cause charge to flow through the conductor at a rate directly proportional to this potential difference, provided that the physical state of the conductor remains unchanged.

If the potential difference across the conductor is increased, there is a proportionate rise in the rate of flow of charge, i.e. the current through the conductor. Such a change occurs within a solid conductor because it is composed of atoms containing a large reserve of electrons, ready to be drawn into forming (increasing) the current. This situation contrasts markedly with the operating conditions of an X-ray tube. Here, electrons are available only in limited quantities. The vacuum has none to offer. The only source is the filament and even here, depending on its temperature, the rate of supply is limited.

It is clear, therefore, that the Ohm's law principle does not control the operation of an X-ray tube. An increase in the kilovoltage across the tube is not accompanied by a proportionate increase in tube current. Instead, the principal factor determining X-ray tube current is the temperature of the filament.

## Saturation

Independence of tube current from the applied kilovoltage is vital to the accuracy of radiographic exposures. It enables the operator of an X-ray generator to choose a tube current (mA) value with confidence, assured that the exposure will not be unexpectedly higher or lower, depending on the influence of the kilovoltage. The situation is made possible by a condition known as saturation.

Students may have met the concept of saturation elsewhere in their previous studies. When an iron or steel specimen is being magnetized, for instance, it eventually reaches a state where all its constituent domains are uniformly aligned. This represents a maximum condition: no amount of extra force will make the specimen more magnetic; it has reached saturation.

Translating this concept to an X-ray tube, where the applied force is the kilovoltage: if, in an experimental situation, the kilovoltage across an X-ray tube were to be set at zero and then gradually increased, the tube current would indeed rise higher and higher, accompanying it – but only until a state had been reached in which electrons were crossing the tube at a rate equal to the rate of their emission from the filament. At this point, because there is no other source of electrons, the rise in current would come to a halt: there would be a state of saturation.

The kilovoltage is thus the cause of the tube current – without its effect, no current would flow – but the maximum achievable tube current is set by the rate at which electrons are being made available by the filament. This rate is, in effect, set by the filament temperature.

X-ray tubes are designed to operate under saturation conditions: the closeness of the electrodes, one to the other; the prescribed range of kilovoltages and filament temperatures; all should ensure that the tube operates under saturation conditions – although in practice the situation may not be ideal, needing some provision of compensation.

## Outline of mA control

An X-ray tube's filament is supplied with a relatively low potential difference, of about 20 V. When applied across the filament, from one end to the other, it causes a current (approximately 3–6 A) to flow through the filament, raising its temperature and causing the emission of electrons.

The low voltage is generated by the tube filament transformer, a step-down transformer whose primary voltage is derived originally from the generator's autotransformer. Since this transformer has a fixed turns ratio,

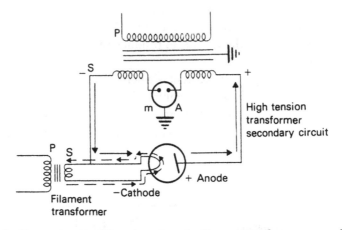

**Fig. 3.1** Tube filament heating. The voltage from the filament transformer causes a heating current to flow through the X-ray tube's filament. During an exposure, electrons flow around the high tension transformer secondary circuit, at a rate controlled by emission from the filament.

its secondary voltage (which is applied across the filament) is controlled by adjustment of the voltage applied across its primary winding. (The same principle is used with the high tension transformer, to control tube kilovoltage.)

The mA control is a form of variable resistor in the primary circuit which supplies voltage to the tube filament transformer. It is adjusted to raise or lower the voltage applied across the transformer's primary winding – so controlling the voltage induced across its secondary winding and applied across the filament.

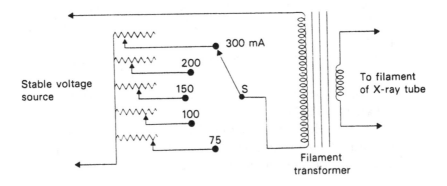

**Fig. 3.2** Tube current selection for radiography. Selector S brings one of the resistors into the circuit, to adjust the voltage applied across the tube filament transformer's primary winding. This is stepped down to the value required for heating the filament to produce the required tube current.

For radiographic exposures, accurate, preset mA values are achieved by a selector which incorporates a *bank* of resistors. Any one of these may be connected into the circuit, to produce the required effect on tube filament heating.

Fluoroscopic tube current – where the effects are immediately visible on the screen – does not require this presetting arrangement. Instead, a continuously variable resistance is provided, allowing slight changes to be made in response to the observed brightness of the screen image.

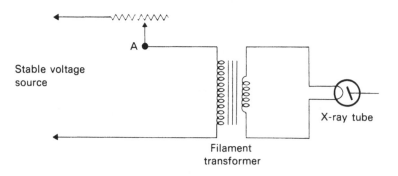

**Fig. 3.3** Tube current selection for fluoroscopy. The selector A adjusts the resistance brought into the circuit, to heat the tube filament to a higher or lower temperature, as required. Adjustment varies the X-ray beam's intensity, in response to the observed brightness of the fluoroscopic image. (This function is usually operated by an automatic monitoring device.)

If a relatively high mA is required, the filament must be raised to a proportionately high operating temperature. This will be achieved by causing a relatively high current to flow through the filament. For a given filament, the means of raising the current is an increase in the voltage applied across it. This is achieved via the transformer, by applying a proportionately high voltage across the primary winding – which is how the mA selector exerts its effect: when set at a high value of resistance, it restricts the voltage applied across the tube filament transformer's primary winding; set at a lower resistance value, it allows the transformer's primary voltage to be higher.

The mA selector thus controls filament temperature and the rate at which the filament emits electrons. Because the tube operates under saturation conditions, the mA selector therefore controls tube current.

### The critical nature of the filament temperature

Tube filament temperature is critical: a relatively small variation away from the correct value can cause a disproportionately large change in tube current

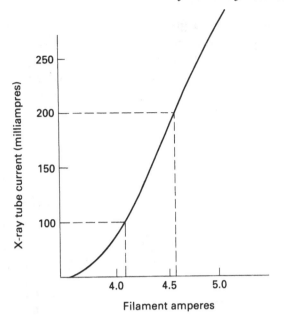

**Fig. 3.4** Relationship between filament current and X-ray tube current. A marked increase in tube current may be produced by a relatively small increase in the filament current. This illustrates the fact that filament temperature is critical: the need for a complex filament heating control circuit is justified.

– and thus in X-ray beam intensity. The electrical supply to the tube filament therefore contains components designed to ensure accuracy in the rate at which electron emission occurs. These will now briefly be considered.

### Voltage stabilizer

Although the voltage induced across each turn of the autotransformer is made independent of mains voltage fluctuations (by the mains voltage compensator), the tube filament supply is in need of even finer control. This device absorbs or cancels out the smallest fluctuations which may occur, even during the exposure itself. This role is performed by the filament voltage stabilizer.

### Space charge compensator

The tube's filament, recessed within its focusing cup, receives some protection from the anode's electric field. This protection allows a small residual cloud of electrons – a small **space charge** – to linger around the filament when the kilovoltage is applied across the tube during an exposure. The strength of the anode's effect varies with kilovoltage, and thus also does its efficiency in attracting electrons out of this protected space charge. At higher kilovoltages, a greater contribution to the tube current from the space charge can be achieved than at lower kilovoltage values.

If left to have its effect, this space charge would spoil the independence which tube current should have from tube kilovoltage: the mA would tend to rise and fall with kV, as a greater or lesser attraction brought electrons across to the anode.

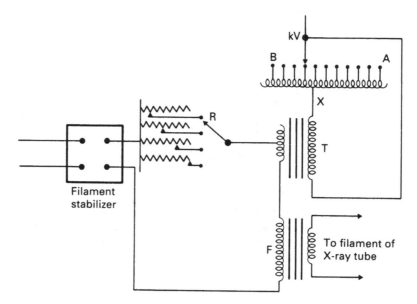

**Fig. 3.5** Space charge compensation. Adjustment of the kilovoltage selector between A and B generates a voltage across the space charge compensator's primary winding, T. This induces a modifying effect on the voltage set by the mA selector, R, for application across the tube filament transformer's primary winding, F.

Instead, a simple compensation device offsets the effect of the space charge, so that tube current is always accurate, whatever the kilovoltage, despite the space charge. The compensator brings a contribution to the filament heating, via the tube filament transformer primary voltage supply.

If a relatively low kilovoltage is selected (which will be less able to attract electrons out of the space charge) a small supplementary voltage is added. This makes the filament slightly hotter so that the actual rate at which electrons are attracted across the tube by that kilovoltage forms exactly the selected tube current.

An interesting consequence of this arrangement may be noticed by observing the maximum safe limits of tube current, at low kilovoltages, as displayed on an X-ray tube rating chart. It would be assumed that, to balance their reduced heating effect on the tube target, low kilovoltages would be usable with the highest mA values. The chart shows otherwise: a cut-off point is marked so that, in effect, higher kilovoltages are indicated as

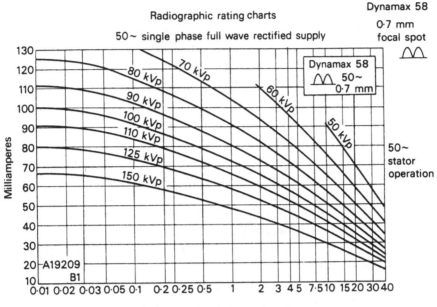

**Fig. 3.6** Space charge compensation. There is a limit to the temperature to which a tube filament can safely be boosted, due to a need to protect the filament from accelerated vaporization. This tube rating chart shows that the maximum tube current allowed when the tube operates at 50 kVp is actually lower than at 100 kVp. (*By courtesy of IGE Medical Systems.*)

safer than lower kilovoltages. The explanation lies in a need to protect the filament (not, in this case, the target) against undue thermal wear. If high mA values were to be produced at these low kilovoltages, the filament temperature boost required (to offset the space charge effect) would be excessive: the filament's life would be unacceptably shortened.

If a relatively high kilovoltage is selected, which will be quite efficient at drawing electrons across the tube from out of the space charge, the tube filament transformer primary voltage is slightly reduced, suppressing the filament temperature, so that the actual rate at which electrons are attracted across the tube is, again, kept at the required, accurate value.

### Ageing of the tube filaments

Tube filaments are made of tungsten, a robust metal with a notably high melting point and low vaporization pressure. It is operated at high temperatures. There is little or no risk that the filament will melt during its operation, but wearing inevitably occurs due to vaporization: atoms of tungsten leave the filament surface, as a result of which the filament becomes thinner. It is in the radiographer's professional interest to minimize this ageing process, by careful use of the tube. It is also in the manufacturers' commercial interests, through their reputation for reliability, to design and incorporate safeguards into their equipment which both delay filament ageing and allow compensation for its effects.

### The filament booster

Between exposures (when the generator is switched on), the tube filament is maintained at a low, stand-by temperature. It is not normally at a full, emission temperature, ready for instantly making an exposure; nor is it kept unheated. This arrangement protects the filament against the full shock of suddenly being heated from *cold* (just as a warm-up procedure protects an anode disc) and restricts the rate of vaporization to a negligibly low level.

The filament booster comprises a resistor in series with the tube filament transformer primary winding, and a bypass switch. The resistor is responsible for the filament being at the low temperature, and not at the high temperature corresponding to the mA setting.

Students will know that, before an exposure is made, a tube has to be *prepared*. Simultaneously with the more obvious anode rotation which occurs, the resistor is short-circuited, allowing the full voltage to be applied across the primary winding of the tube filament transformer, raising the tube filament to its full emission temperature.

By this arrangement, the period of maximum wear is restricted to the duration of the exposure, preceded by the short tube preparation time. Radiographers can play their part in assisting this safety provision, by delaying tube preparation until just before the exposure is to be made.

### Trimming resistors

Despite careful use, a tube filament inevitably becomes thinner as a result of vaporization. There is thus a reduction in both its surface area and its cross-sectional area. The reduced surface area lessens its emission capability, while the reduction in cross-sectional area increases its electrical resistance. For a fixed voltage, an increase in resistance reduces the current and thus also the temperature rise, leading to a further drop in emission.

Compensatory resistors are built in to the filament transformer supply circuits, to offset this wearing. Their values are reduced as required, when periodic service checks are made on the accuracy of the preselected mA values. In this way, by a compensatory increase in filament temperature, as it ages, required rates of electron emission are sustained throughout the life of a tube.

*Tube filament transformers*

Each tube filament has its own supply. As well as having differing physical characteristics (length, diameter, wire thickness) each filament will tend to wear at a different rate, depending on how regularly it is used. The *broad* and *fine* filaments are therefore each supplied from a separate transformer and there is a focus selector, changeover switch to energize one or the other, depending on radiographic need.

Through their connection to the X-ray tube's cathode, the tube filament transformers' secondary windings are at high tension. These transformers therefore need the shockproofing provided for all components in the HT circuit. They are thus located with the high tension transformer in its tank.

**High tension connections**

The tube filament transformers provide secondary output voltages to be applied across the tube filaments. Despite the appearances suggested by circuit diagrams, there may be a considerable distance between transformers and tube. In the case of single tank construction, the transformers can be adjacent to the tube insert. More usually, however, there is a distance bridged by the HT cables. The cables' central conductors carry the tube current but also conduct the filament heating currents. For this purpose, there are usually three conductors: each of the two filaments having its separate connection, while the third, shared or common conductor is employed for the filament currents and tube current.

## 3.4 *Falling load* generators

Old types of X-ray generator offer the user a free choice of the tube current values within the limits of X-ray tube safety. Usually, fixed, preset values – 100 mA, 200 mA, 300 mA, etc. – for radiography; and a continuously variable tube current for fluoroscopic (and possibly tomographic) purposes.

Modern generators tend to offer their users (either directly or via an anatomical programme) selection of mAs, rather than identified tube currents. In these instances, selection of optimal mA and exposure time combinations (within the tube's rating) is made by a computer, possibly together with an automatic exposure control device. This may involve a *falling load* method of mA selection.

Conventionally, restrictions may be imposed on the usefulness of relatively high values of mA by the shortness of the exposure times for which they can be safely used. This limitation arises from a preconception that an mAs value must be the product of an exposure time and a fixed mA. The falling load principle allows an exposure to be regarded more flexibly:

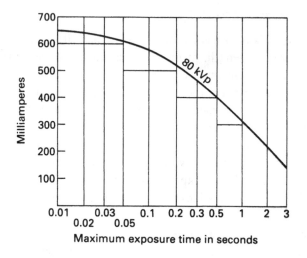

**Fig. 3.7** The *falling load* principle. A required value of mAs may be achieved as a succession of exposure increments, each, in turn, at a reduced mA value:

$$600\,\text{mA} \times 0.05\,\text{s} = \phantom{0}30$$
$$500\,\text{mA} \times 0.15\,\text{s} = \phantom{0}75$$
$$400\,\text{mA} \times 0.3\,\text{s} \phantom{0}= 120$$
$$300\,\text{mA} \times 0.5\,\text{s} \phantom{0}= \underline{150}$$
$$375\,\text{mAs}$$

By this arrangement, tube current is gradually reduced, to match the X-ray tube's *characteristic* or its declining capacity (as heat accumulates), so enabling exposure times to be minimal. Note the similarity to an X-ray tube rating chart.

as an unbroken sequence of separate increments, each with a different tube current, falling with the safe availability of mA, within tube rating. The practical benefit of the falling load principle is that exposures tend to be delivered within the shortest times available – with proportionate reduction in the risk of image movement unsharpness.

During a falling load exposure, there will be a reduction – either continuous or stepped – in tube filament heating, as the exposure progresses. Selection and control will thus be automatic rather than manual.

## 3.5 Tube current measurement and display

Whereas X-ray tube kilovoltage is displayed on a generator control panel indirectly by a calibrated device, because it cannot feasibly be measured

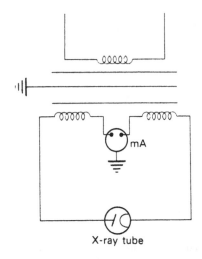

**Fig. 3.8** mA indication. An mA indicator (meter) is connected in series with the X-ray tube so that it may conduct the tube current. The indicator is sited at the earthed midpoint of the high tension transformer's secondary winding, so that it can safely be included on the generator's control panel.

actually across the tube, tube current can be directly measured. The principle of current measurement – that the measuring device must be in series connection within the circuit – can be applied, even though the X-ray tube is at a high kilovoltage with respect to earth potential.

The fact which makes this possible is that the midpoint of the HT transformer's secondary winding is at earth potential. This arrangement, designed to reduce insulation requirements in the HT circuit, coincidentally provides a site for a tube current measuring device which can safely be placed on the generator control panel. Because it is in series with the tube, despite being physically separated from it, across a room (despite the closeness falsely implied by a circuit diagram), this device can actually record tube current, and show whether it is correct or incorrect.

A common situation where measurement may prove difficult is when the duration of the exposure is too brief to allow the mA measuring device to respond to the tube current. When this is the case, a device which measures mAs – that is, the electric charge which crosses the tube during the exposure – rather the rate at which charge flows, can be employed. This then gives a reading in proportion to the quantity of radiation produced and provides a check on tube current and exposure time accuracy. Some generators may provide simultaneous display of both mA and mAs. Otherwise, the changeover from current to charge reading will be an automatic function, depending on the exposure factors selected.

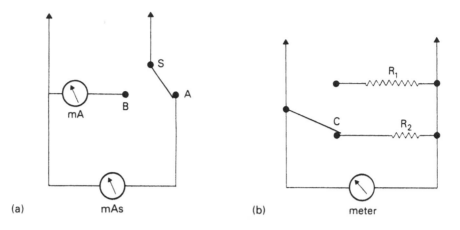

**Fig. 3.9** Indication of mA and mAs. (a) Short exposures may be recorded more accurately by an mAs indicator (meter) than an mA indicator. Switch S makes a series connection between the X-ray tube and either (at A) the mAs, or (at B) the mA indicator. Switching may be automatically made when exposure time is selected. (b) If a meter is used for mA or mAs indication, it may, for improved accuracy, have a low range scale (full-scale deflection) as well as the high range scale. Automatic changeover of contact C brings either R1 or R2 into the circuit, to provide a scale appropriate to a particular exposure.

## 3.6 Follow-up practical

Carry out a survey of the X-ray generators to which you have access within your clinical imaging department.

(1) What mA values (ranges) are available from each generator? How do these – particularly the maximum values – relate to the types of rectification (tube kV supply waveform) provided by the generator?

(2) Find out whether selection of a particular tube current (mA) for radiography is available, or only mAs (milliampere second) values. If there is no facility at all for selecting mA or mAs, is this linked to an *anatomical programme*?

(3) Try to discover why variation of mA/mAs selection exists across the range of generators: is this random, as a result of recent purchasing, or matched to the radiographic (clinical) functions of each generator?

(4) Ask experienced members of staff which of the generators they prefer to operate – or which they dislike!

# Chapter 4
# Exposure Timing and Switching

## 4.1 Introduction

As technological advances have raised achievable X-ray tube current values and increased the speed of image recording media, the average radiographic exposure time has become shorter. This reduction has brought an increased need for accuracy of exposure timing: margins for error virtually no longer exist. Consequently, the only type of (manual selection) exposure timer now used in X-ray equipment is the *electronic*, and this itself has become miniaturized into what engineers regard, if it ever becomes faulty, as a disposable item.

As users of this very reliable and, in practice, unmendable device, student radiographers no longer need to occupy themselves with learning its detailed circuitry. The simple principles of the electronic timer are useful, however, as an introduction to studying a type over which radiographers can exercise some control: the automatic exposure timer – although this itself is increasingly becoming part of computer selected anatomical programmes.

Similarly, exposure switching is reliable: electronic circuitry has replaced electromechanical devices. The action of safety interlocks, which protect an X-ray tube by blocking the use of exposure factors which will cause damage, are also increasingly being taken out of the radiographer's routine responsibility. In that their action has a bearing on a student's comprehension of tube operation, however, a brief description of these will be included.

This chapter will therefore outline, rather than exhaustively describe, exposure timing and switching.

## 4.2 Exposure switching

Radiographic exposures begin when a voltage is applied across the primary winding of the HT transformer. Immediately, the required kilovoltage is induced across the secondary winding, rectified and applied across the tube, to produce X-rays.

The exposure switch, with which all student radiographers become familiar, is not the actual switch which closes in the transformer's primary circuit. Instead, it sends an impulse to two electronic switches: responsible for (a) starting the exposure and (b) starting the exposure timer.

At the end of the exposure, the primary circuit is re-opened by a signal from the exposure timer.

Two technical problems complicate switching in the primary circuit. First, the current has a high value, which makes it more difficult than switching a low current; and the other concerns the fact that the current is alternating. Addressing this second point lessens the difficulty of the first. If it can be arranged that switching – both on and off – coincides with points during the alternating cycle when the instantaneous value is zero, damage to the switch is less likely. This arrangement also ensures that the exposure time occupies an exact number of half-cycles of the supply voltage (the number being determined by the exposure timer). In doing so, however, the minimum exposure time is one half of a cycle.

To obtain exposure times which are shorter than a half-cycle – such as are required by rapid serial techniques, for example – switching may be performed without the convenience of phasing to zero points. Alternatively, exposures may be switched in the HT secondary circuit. Here the technical problem is not presented by the magnitude of the current – usually less than 1 A – but by the high voltages.

One method by which secondary switching may be managed is by an arrangement concerning the X-ray tube itself. For normal operation, electron emission from the filament is formed into a controlled beam by the application of a negative potential to the cathode's focusing cup. The application of an even higher potential can actually block emission of electrons altogether, and thus prevent the production of X-rays from the anode. The switching of X-ray exposures – on and off – is thus achievable by the release and reapplication of a sufficiently high negative potential or **bias** to block electron escape from the cathode. Meanwhile, electrons continue to be emitted from the filament but to no effect. This cathode switching requires modified electrical connections to the X-ray tube via an HT cable which incorporates an extra conductor.

## 4.3 Exposure timing

### Principle of the electronic timer

There are three principal components:

- A capacitor;
- A selection of resistors; and
- A voltage-sensitive *trigger* switching device.

When a potential difference is connected across a capacitor, electric charges begin to accumulate on its plates. The quantity of charge on the plates rises to a value dependent on the capacitor's capacitance and the applied potential difference (voltage). Growth in the quantity of charge ceases when the potential difference rises to equal the external, applied voltage.

An important feature of this phenomenon is that the time taken for charging to occur is predictable. It depends on two factors: the capacitance of the capacitor (that is, the quantity of charge it stores per unit potential difference) and the resistance of the conducting path via which the external potential difference is applied.

If capacitance and resistance are constant, the charging time of a capacitor up to a given voltage is accurately reproducible. If the resistance of the conducting path is increased, the charging time is proportionately increased. In other words, the time taken to charge a capacitor can be controlled by adjustment of the resistance through which it charges.

A voltage-sensitive trigger switch will operate when the potential difference applied across it rises to a predetermined value. Below this value, the switch remains open; at and above the critical value, the switch closes.

Such a trigger switch is employed in an electronic timer, to end radiographic exposures. The voltage across it is applied from a capacitor. Before an exposure is made, the capacitor is discharged (zero volts) and the switch is open.

When an exposure time is selected, an appropriate resistor is brought into the circuit via which the capacitor will be charged. Charging does not begin until the exposure switch starts the exposure. When this is activated (when the radiographer *exposes*) charge flows through the circuit onto the capacitor's plates, charging it up towards the critical value at which the trigger will operate to end the exposure.

The time taken for this to occur depends on the value of the resistance through which the capacitor is charging. Thus, by variation of the resistance, control can be exercised over exposure times.

When a radiographer preselects a particular exposure time, therefore, what happens electrically is that a resistor of an appropriate value (small for short times, large for long) is connected into the circuit, to determine whether the capacitor will charge quickly or slowly, i.e. whether the end of the exposure will be early or delayed.

Another form of exposure timer is actually able to count the voltage pulses applied across the X-ray tube during the exposure. This facility can be used to produce (and accurately reproduce) the very shortest exposure times.

*Automatic exposure timers*

### Introduction

For many years, accurate and consistent manual preselection of the quantity of X-radiation required for any given image (the product of tube current and exposure time) has represented a constant difficulty for diagnostic radiographers. Unpredictable opacities within the anatomical region being examined can surprise even the most experienced operators.

Surveys conducted on a wide scale have drawn the conclusion that inaccurate exposures have been the most common cause for radiographs needing to be repeated. The consequences of this malpractice are clear to all, including the patient concerned: a doubling of the radiation hazard, the costs and the time; the emotional stresses on the patient ('Why did they want *another* one?') and the inconvenience imposed on other patients who are waiting to receive the radiographer's attention.

Automatic radiograph processing and equipment reliability now leave inaccurate exposure selection starkly open to scrutiny as a malpractice which is all the more regrettable because, in most cases, it can be avoided.

### Principle of automatic exposure timing

An automatic exposure device monitors the beam of X-rays transmitted through the part of the patient's body which is being examined, and terminates the exposure when a sufficient quantity of radiation has been received to produce a radiographic image of the required density.

It could be mentioned that although the purpose of these automatic devices is to exercise accurate control on the quantity of radiation, their method is almost invariably to achieve this by influencing exposure time – and for this reason they are usually known as automatic exposure timers, or autotimers.

Measurement of the transmitted X-ray beam is achieved by employing either of two properties of X-rays: ionization or fluorescence. Accordingly, there are two distinct types of device: termed **ionization chamber timers** and **photoelectric timers**. Ionization timers are normally to be found in radiographic equipment while phototimers, which operate through the action of light from a fluorescent screen, are normally to be found incorporated in fluorographic equipment.

It should be noted that there are extreme situations in which the required exposure times are too short – a few milliseconds – for autotimers to operate reliably. In these instances, preset exposure times are used.

### Ionization chamber timers

These employ very thin, plastic-walled, radiolucent chambers located between the patient and the film. When irradiated, ionization occurs within the chamber, the ions are attracted towards the electrodes (of the opposite sign) and a current flows. The voltage applied across the chamber is set at a value which will ensure that saturation will occur: ions will be collected before they can recombine, so that the current will accurately represent X-ray intensity.

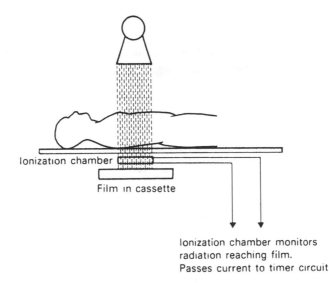

Ionization chamber

Film in cassette

Ionization chamber monitors
radiation reaching film.
Passes current to timer circuit

**Fig. 4.1** Ionization chamber type automatic exposure timer. Location of the chamber in relation to the patient and the film.

This ionization current (rather than one flowing through a preselected resistance) is employed, after passing through an amplification process, to charge a capacitor – as in an electronic timer – and terminate the exposure when it has reached a critical voltage.

The arrangement thus produces exposure times which are proportional to the need imposed by the object's radiopacity. If the object is relatively opaque (large, dense), the intensity of the transmitted X-ray beam will tend to be low. Ionization caused by this transmitted beam will occur at a proportionately low rate, giving rise to a low current which charges the capacitor slowly, giving a long exposure time.

If, on the other hand, the object is relatively radiolucent (thin, easily penetrated), the transmitted X-ray beam will be intense. Ionization will occur at a high rate, the current will be high and swift charging will bring the exposure to an early conclusion.

For general use, automatic exposure timing equipment tends to incorporate more than one chamber. This extends its anatomical usefulness and reliability. The usual arrangement is for three chambers to be incorporated within a radiolucent assembly which is positioned between the patient and the film. (If a grid is being used, the chamber lies between the grid and the film.)

Selection of chambers is made according to the anatomical structures which make up the imaging field and their significance as typical, reliable guides to an accurate image density. They are sometimes referred to as *dominant* areas.

To illustrate their use: if an anteroposterior projection of the vertebral column is being exposed, the chamber which is located centrally – coinciding with the central position of the vertebral column – will be

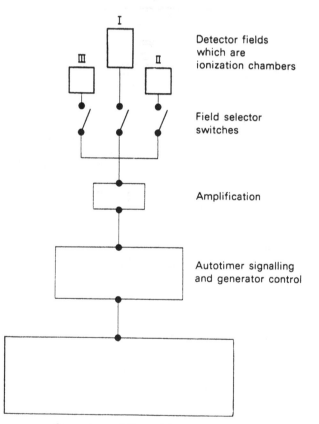

Fig. 4.2 Ionization chambers in an automatic exposure timer. Fields (chambers) are selected according to the anatomical structures to be included on the radiograph. Ionization currents need to be amplified before use in determining exposure times.

employed for monitoring the radiation intensity transmitted through the patient. If a postero-anterior projection of the adult chest is being exposed, a chamber which aligns to an area of the lung fields will be selected as representative of the whole of the thorax. This will occupy an offcentred position, usually termed a *lateral* chamber.

Timer controls allow the radiographer to preset the quantity of radiation required before the exposure will be terminated. In effect, this is the value which will produce a correctly exposed radiograph, but there is an important link between these two criteria. This principally involves the photographic speed of the film and intensifying screens which are used, in given circumstances, to convert the radiation pattern into a radiographic image. The control offered to the radiographer is, therefore, designated as an image density selector – usually as a short range of plus or minus values, about a basic average. In practice, since the *useful density range* of most radiographs tends to be fairly common, little variation may be required.

## Practical operation

Correct use of an automatic timer for radiography involves a set procedure which must be carefully followed:

**(1)** *Selection of chamber(s)*. These, as has been mentioned, are determined by the anatomical region and the radiographic projection being taken.

**(2)** *Selection of density*. This is normally according to a predetermined value, based on experience for a given radiographic projection. Care must be taken that the value relates exactly to the selected chamber(s) and the film/screen speed being used.

**(3)** *Correction factor for radiation quality*. The chamber's response does not vary linearly with radiation quality. The timer controls may include correction factors to select if the tube kilovoltage exceeds specified values, e.g. 90 kV or 120 kV, and/or correction factors which take into account the filtration variation created by the size of the object (possibly expressed as patient build).

**(4)** *Accurate positioning of the patient*. It is important that the patient is positioned accurately in relation to the site of the ionization chamber. If the anatomical parts aligned to the chamber are more radiolucent or more opaque than normal, due to inaccurate positioning, the image density will be less or more than it should be.

**(5)** *Primary beam collimation*. Standardization of collimation will tend to minimize the variable influence upon radiation measurement of the scatter emitted from the patient, and thus upon image density.

**(6)** *Allowance for known pathology*. If the selected, dominant anatomical area has had its radiopacity altered by pathological changes, the exposure time and resulting image density will be appropriate to this situation. This is, after all, one of the benefits of automated exposure control. If, however, an image density is required which is appropriate to some other area within the area being examined, another chamber should be used and the selected density value adjusted accordingly.

(7) *Setting of the control panel time to an excess value.* If the autotimer develops a fault which affects its ability to terminate the exposure, the *normal* manually preselected time set on the generator console will operate, to prevent the potentially serious consequences (to the patient and the X-ray tube) of a continuing exposure. In this role, the ordinary timer is acting as a *guard* timer.

It is important, however, that the ordinary timer is set to a value which slightly exceeds the expected autotimed value. If it is set to a shorter time, the ordinary timer – not the autotimer – will operate, resulting in an underexposed image.

**Phototimers**

These are normally employed in equipment such as a fluorographic camera, which operates through the creation of some form of fluorescent light image. The sensory part of the timer tends to be more complicated than an ionization chamber. For this reason it has tended, in direct radiography, to be positioned behind the cassette, where unfortunately detection is less reliable than in front. Newer designs, however, incorporate radiolucent material which can generate fluorescent light and, by a fibre-optic action, convey it to circuitry lying outside the path of the primary beam.

The principle is parallel to the ionization chamber type, in that measurement of X-ray intensity takes place during the exposure until a predetermined point is reached. In this case, a photodetector device monitors the brightness of a fluorescent light image created by the X-rays emerging from the patient. This device emits electrons – and therefore permits conduction of charge – in direct proportion to the intensity of visible light incident upon it. In other words, its resistance becomes lower and the current through it becomes greater, as light intensity increases. This current tends to be very low, however, and requires amplification (photomultiplication) before it can be used to charge the capacitor in the timer circuit.

Again, the automation relationships are easy to appreciate. If the anatomical area is relatively radiopaque (thick, dense), the fluorescent image will tend to be rather dim, in proportion to the low intensity of emergent X-rays. The photodetector will generate a relatively low current, taking a long time to charge the capacitor and terminate the exposure.

If the anatomical area is more radiolucent (thin, easily penetrated), the emergent X-ray beam will have a high intensity. It will create a relatively bright fluorescent image, and the proportionately high current which it causes will bring the exposure to an early termination.

Phototimers may monitor a whole image, rather than selected dominant areas, and their use therefore tends to be more automated (when compared with the ionization chamber type).

### *Exposure interlocks*

To assume that an exposure can be made simply because tube kilovoltage, current and exposure time have been set as required, overlooks the possibility that it may not be safe to make such an exposure.

An interlock is a device which links two or more functions together, to ensure that they take place safely in a correct order. A common, everyday example is found in household appliances such as a microwave oven or a tumble dryer: the door must be firmly closed before the magnetron or the electric motor will operate.

Interlocks are to be found in many radiographic situations. Some concern physical or radiation safety. Those which are designed to protect the X-ray tube, allowing or preventing an X-ray exposure, may be considered in two groups.

First, there are those which are designed to ensure that before an exposure takes place, the filament has been boosted to its full emission temperature and the anode has achieved its correct rotational speed. These may be simply time delay devices rather than true interlocks.

The second group operate according to the projected amount of heat, or the rate at which the heat will be produced, accompanying X-ray production during the exposure. Computed calculations of heat production are compared with the safe heat capacities of the X-ray tube – not only the absolute values but also with regard to the present temperature, to take account of residual heat from previous exposures.

Any attempts to set kV, mA and exposure time values which would prove unsafe are blocked. On the console of an older, manually controlled generator, this situation would illuminate a warning to the operator to revise the settings. A modern, automatic generator goes straight to the stage of setting safe factors, leaving the radiographer free to concentrate on matters which defy automation.

## 4.4 Follow-up practical

Anatomical programming, with automation of timing and switching functions, may leave the student little scope to investigate timer operation. However:

(1) Make a study of the practical steps taken to ensure that the autotimers used for radiography actually perform their role accurately. What aspects of technique (e.g. centring, density selection, collimation) are critical to success, i.e. the correct exposure of every radiograph?

(2) What tests are carried out to check the accurate, consistent operation of an autotimer, and what action is taken if the timer's calibration and settings are suspected of being faulty?

(3) Manually set timers can be tested: most routinely by the convenience of an electronic *box* but also, if available, by some form of *spinning top*.
Historically, a spinning top was a manually (and very variably) propelled device, recording dot images of the discrete X-ray pulses produced by a single-phase generator. Opportunities for performing this test may, therefore, be rare.
The successor to this device may be found still in use: an electrically driven, constant velocity top which checks exposure times by the sector or angle through which it passes during an exposure. This can be used whatever the tube's supply waveform. It may be possible to perform tests in parallel, to investigate their accuracy, as well as that of the timer.

(4) The use of a *grid* X-ray tube for rapid, secondary switching may be investigated, if circumstances allow.

# Part Three
# General and Multipurpose Radiographic Equipment

X-ray imaging is practised with the aim of producing maximum diagnostic information from a minimum amount of radiation. In universal use, therefore, are devices which confine the X-ray field to the smallest size needed to demonstrate a required anatomical area. This limitation, as well as protecting the patient, tends to enhance image contrast, by reducing the amount of scattered radiation reaching the imaging area (film or screen). Supplementary to this action is the role of an anti-scatter grid. Control of scatter is the principal subject of Chapter 5.

Almost every imaging department includes what may be known as its *general X-ray room*. These are versatile; within them can be performed a wide range of radiographic examinations, through the simplicity of their equipment: a freely moveable X-ray tube and a multipurpose radiographic couch or vertical stand.

Chapter 6 takes a look at these basic items, both for their own importance and so that comparisons can be drawn between them and the specialized equipment covered in later chapters. Even within the limits of the facilities they provide, there are many styles and designs. It would be impossible to describe all these or to keep up with innovations. Instead, the key features are covered and readers are asked to see these applied in practice, for themselves.

# Chapter 5
# Control of Scattered X-Radiation

## 5.1 Introduction

When an X-ray beam encounters an object, three phenomena can occur:

(1) *The X-ray photons can pass through unhindered*. When a patient is radiographed, these photons are responsible for creating the exposed parts of the image: densities on a conventional radiograph; and the brighter areas of a fluoroscopic image.

(2) *Photons can be absorbed by the object*. Absorption is the process in which energy is transferred from the X-ray beam to the object, and is clearly a major focus of interest when radiation protection is being studied. Concerning the radiographic image: the elimination of photons from the beam is responsible for the areas of lesser exposure: lower densities on a radiograph and darker areas of a fluoroscopic image, which complement more fully exposed areas, to form a total image.

(3) *Photons can interact with the object* in such a way that their progress continues – but in a different direction. These photons are said to have been **scattered**. In contrast to the **primary radiation** which emanates directly from the X-ray tube, scattered radiation is classified as **secondary radiation**.

## 5.2 The effects of scattered radiation

In diagnostic radiography, scattered radiation has two potential effects:

(1) Travelling out of an irradiated object in all directions, it can pose a **radiation hazard** to personnel nearby. By spreading within the body of the irradiated patient, it can carry the ionizing effects of the radiation to parts distant from the area being investigated, which ought strictly to remain free from exposure. Such internal spread cannot totally be avoided but ought to be minimized, particularly where structures of greater radio-sensitivity are involved.

(2) Scatter travelling in a direction towards the X-ray film or image intensifier can also increase image density, adding to the effects of the primary radiation, but in a random manner: it carries no useful information about the object's shape and composition; its effect is to *reduce image contrast*.

## 5.3 Methods of scatter control

The harmful and undesirable effects of scattered radiation can be lessened in two distinct ways:

(1) The amount of scattered radiation *actually produced* during an exposure can be reduced. This is achieved by minimizing the volume of tissue exposed to the primary beam. Routine reduction of the cross-sectional area of the aperture through which the primary beam passes is the major method by which this volume of tissue is minimized. This action is termed collimation.

Effectiveness of collimation is strongly dependent on the accuracy with which the X-ray beam is centred to the anatomical area of interest. If centring is inaccurate, collimation carries the risk ultimately of increasing the hazard to the patient, by excluding some significant surrounding structures from the image field.

Reduction in the volume of exposed tissue can also be achieved, in limited circumstances, by reducing the path of the primary beam (rather than its cross-section) by some form of compression device, which, more properly, achieves tissue displacement.

Table 5.1 Comparison between methods of enhancing radiographic image contrast.

| *Primary beam collimation* | *Use of a secondary radiation grid* |
| --- | --- |
| Reduces the radiation dose to the patient | *Increases* the dose to the patient, due to the fact that an increased exposure is needed – to compensate for the absorbed primary radiation |
| Has no effect on image unsharpness | May increase image unsharpness – both movement and geometric |
| May reduce hazard to staff | May increase hazard to staff |
| Simple to use | May be complicated to use correctly |

(2) Scatter which leaves the irradiated object can be absorbed before it creates its undesired, external effect. In the case of presenting a hazard to nearby personnel, this absorption is achieved simply by placing substantial protective barriers in the path of the scatter.

In the case of the image-recording device, the task of absorbing scatter is complicated by the need, simultaneously, to allow primary, image-forming X-rays to pass unhindered. This selective action, distinguishing between primary and scattered radiation, is routinely achieved by the use of a grid.

## X-ray beam centring devices

Since the importance of correct centring is related closely to beam collimation, it is usual to find that a single device serves both purposes. In some situations, however, the collimator gives little or no assistance to the radiographer in centring the beam to the object. In these cases – where the beam is collimated by a single plate diaphragm, for example – some form of illuminated, centre-indicating device may be fitted.

## X-ray beam collimators

### Cone
Students may still find examples of this traditional device in use, although its shortcomings have led to its virtual disappearance from general radiography, despite its simple benefits.

A cone is in the form of a metal cylinder which clips or screws onto a socket mounted surrounding the X-ray tube port. Cones can be short, long or telescopic; parallel-sided or tapered; and circular or rectangular in cross-section. They produce X-ray fields of predictable and reproducible shape and size, for techniques where standardization, and possibly an irregular field shape, are required. Shortcomings lie in their lack of adjustment and usually a poor indication of beam centring.

### Light beam diaphragm (LBD)
The LBD is fitted as a standard accessory to most X-ray tubes used for diagnostic techniques. Collimation is achieved by sets of symmetrically positioned, adjustable metal plates or **leaves** which surround a central channel through which the X-ray beam passes. The leaves are adjusted in towards or out, away from the centre, as required. In opposing pairs, the leaves are hinged to move on a rigid frame which is enclosed in a metal box housing. Movement of the leaves is controlled by knobs or levers, outside the housing. These controls indicate field sizes at given distances, by

movement along calibrated scales. The side of the housing remote from the X-ray tube is mostly formed by a transparent plastic window.

The accuracy and popularity of this device, which has led to its standardized use, arises from incorporation of an electric lamp and a radiolucent mirror. The lamp is mounted towards the edge of the housing, out of the path of the X-ray beam. Its light shines onto the mirror which is mounted precisely along the central axis of the X-ray beam, at an angle of 45°. From here, the mirror reflects light from the lamp exactly along the path of the X-ray beam, out of the housing via its transparent window. Movement of the leaves widens or narrows the light beam and the field size it casts on the radiographic object. It thus indicates to the radiographer the field size and shape which will be formed when an X-ray exposure is made.

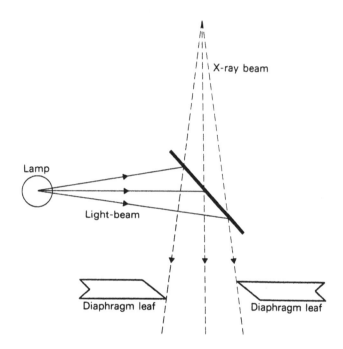

**Fig. 5.1** Principle of a light beam diaphragm. Note the equal distances between the tube target (source of X-rays) and the mirror, and between the light source and the mirror. The mirror is set at 45° to the central X-ray. The closing edges of the diaphragm leaves are chamfered obliquely, to overlap when the aperture is closed, to form a continuous barrier against the X-rays, for safety.

The benefits of an LBD are:

(1) a visible demonstration of beam centring and the field shape and size; and

(2) an infinite variety of field size and shape, giving the opportunity of optimum protection and image contrast, in all situations.

The leaves of a standard LBD give a rectangular field. This matches the shape of X-ray films. Some other LBDs have sickle-shaped leaves arranged as an iris, to produce a circular X-ray field, which may form a better match for the shape of some anatomical structures, notably the skull. A few LBDs offer both rectangular and circular fields.

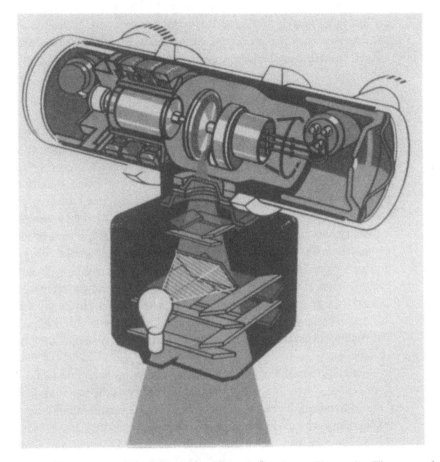

**Fig. 5.2** Sectioned display of a light beam diaphragm fitted to an X-ray tube. Three sets of leaves, working in synchronization, collimate the field, with sharp edges, free from penumbra. (*By courtesy of Siemens plc.*)

The limitations of an LBD become obvious when the lamp fails or the mirror is dislodged from its precise position. The lamp has to produce an intense light, to compete with daylight and room lighting conditions. Despite modern lamp technology, the time comes when a lamp fails and the operator has no light beam to indicate field size and centring. Having a replacement lamp ready to hand is the surest remedy in this situation, together with knowledge of how to remove the old lamp and fit the new. Careful, sparing use of the lamp – only during centring and collimating of the beam – is a wise precaution to lessen the occurrence of failures. Most LBDs have a timed switch–off device fitted, to guard against forgetfulness. As well as needlessly ageing the lamp, prolonged overuse can raise the temperature of the LBD housing, increasing its chance of inflicting a skin burn, when touched.

Gentle handling of the X-ray tube and LBD will tend to keep the device operating accurately but, even so, regular checks are advisable as part of a quality assurance programme. Commercial test equipment is available but locally constructed devices, based on the same principles, can be equally effective.

## Test for LBD accuracy

To check coincidence of light and X-ray beams, a test exposure on an X-ray film is needed. The tube is centred to a film and a field size set within the film's perimeter, allowing a 2–3 cm margin. Metallic or other radiopaque markers are placed at the corners of the light field, together with an indication of the field's orientation to the X-ray tube (to show anode end, etc.). Two exposures are made. The first uses the marked settings, to create a density showing the limits of the X-ray field. The second is a smaller exposure, with the field widened to include the whole film. This is a precaution to show the opaque markers, even if there is a deviation which excludes them from the first radiation field. To detect the chance of an error caused by free movement of the mirror, the test should be performed with the tube both horizontal and vertical. A variation of 1% is normally acceptable; thus, a 1 cm error at a focus–film distance of 1 m may be overlooked.

Accurate operation of an LBD depends on its correct attachment to the X-ray tube. This is originally the responsibility of the installation engineers. Careful handling by radiographers needs to be supplemented by occasional inspection, to confirm a secure fit. Alignment of the LBD to the centre of the tube port can be measured by a type of sighting device which incorporates a small, metallic ball bearing and a slightly larger metallic ring or washer. Correct alignment produces concentric images of these two objects.

Student radiographers must recognize the illusion of smallness which a light field can create when it is separated, along the path of the beam, from the film plane. The illuminated field – on a patient's abdominal wall, for example – may suggest inadequacy of film coverage, due to the divergent geometry of the beam. This must not prompt readjustment to a larger size (for fear of 'missing something off') to expose areas outside the film's margins. The introduction by manufacturers of automatic cassette size sensors, with feedback to diaphragm controls, is a welcome safeguard against the dangers of inaccuracy.

## *Elimination of scatter from the emergent X-ray beam*

### Principle of a grid

Students will recognize that elimination of scatter is only one of the functions of a grid; it also has to allow transmission of primary radiation. Discrimination between the two is achieved according to their different directions of travel. Whereas primary radiation travels along predictable, straight lines from the X-ray tube's target, scattered photons travel in random directions.

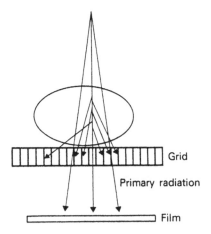

Fig. 5.3 Principle of an anti-scatter grid. Primary X-radiation is transmitted through the aligned spaces between the parallel opaque strips, shown here in section. Oblique scatter fails to pass through these interspaces, being absorbed by the opaque strips. (It must be brought to the reader's attention that this diagram has been selectively drawn for its purpose. In reality, also, some primary radiation is absorbed by the opaque strips, and some scatter passes unhindered through the interspaces.)

The key material included in a grid is lead. This is incorporated into the grid as extremely thin strips, end-on to the approaching primary radiation. They thus absorb the minimum of primary and form the opaque walls of channels through which the primary will pass with little or no absorption. This transmission of primary is achieved through alignment of the radiolucent channels to the predictable path of the primary beam.

Scattered radiation has no predictable path, beyond the likelihood that it will deviate from the direction of the primary. It will thus tend to approach a grid at angles which do not align with the clear path through the radiolucent channels. Travelling along such paths, it will tend to encounter the lead strips, where it will be absorbed and fail to be transmitted through to form an image.

## Types of grid

The simplest type of grid is composed of a series of precisely parallel lead strips, supported and held exactly in their places by a radiolucent material such as plastic, aluminium or carbon fibre. This type, usually termed a *parallel* grid, is relatively simple to manufacture and offers the benefits of simplicity. It can be used satisfactorily in circumstances where a cassette is in a free position, not aligned to the middle of a couch or vertical bucky stand, where accurate centring of the X-ray beam to the grid cannot be easily achieved.

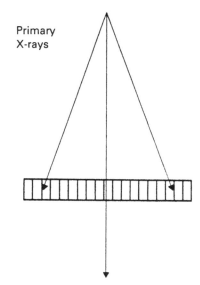

Primary
X-rays

**Fig. 5.4** Primary beam absorption by a parallel grid. Towards its lateral margins, misalignment between oblique X-rays and the parallel spaces reduces the transmitted intensity.

The main shortcoming of a parallel grid is that, away from its centre line, there is an increasing misalignment between the parallel, radiolucent spaces and the divergent X-ray beam. This leads to a reduction in the transmitted primary beam intensity which may be observed as a tendency, along these lateral margins, for images to be underexposed.

The problem of misalignment is solved by positioning of the lead strips so that, while still basically parallel, they are tilted slightly in towards the midline, so that the radiolucent spaces match the angles at which the diverging primary beam approaches. This arrangement forms the principle of a *focused* grid.

The advantage of freer primary transmission is offset by the need for use of a focused grid to be more critical: the user must take care that there actually is alignment between the divergent rays and the oblique,

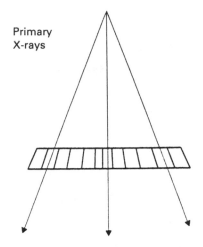

Primary
X-rays

**Fig. 5.5** Principle of grid focusing. Oblique tilting of the lead strips creates interspaces aligned to the diverging primary beam. This allows maximum intensity of primary transmission, across the full width of the grid. Note the need for coincidence between the position of the tube's focal spot and the grid's focal centre.

radiolucent grid interspaces. This requires accurate centring of the X-ray beam to the grid's midline, and use at the correct focus–grid distance. Focused grids are manufactured and clearly marked for use at prescribed focus–grid distances. These are matched to the usual focus–film distances employed in diagnostic radiography. Use of other distances, either longer or shorter than the precise length, leads to a tendency for primary beam absorption to increase at the grid's lateral margins. In practice, some tolerance or latitude is permissible, but this should be minimized by the user.

The action of the lead strips is to absorb X-radiation travelling transversely across a grid. The purpose is to absorb scattered radiation, but any primary radiation travelling in this same direction will similarly be absorbed. One restriction on a grid's use, therefore, (whether parallel or focused) is that transverse X-ray beam angulations are prohibited. If the X-ray beam is to be angled, this must be *along* the grid, rather than *across*.

This freedom to angle the primary beam highlights a deficiency in the grid's ability to absorb scattered radiation: any scatter which happens to travel along the axis of a radiolucent channel will be transmitted freely through to affect the image. In most situations, this failure on the grid's part to absorb some scatter is tolerable. There may be other occasions, however, where scatter is produced in such large quantities (during simultaneous biplane exposures, for example) and may have a proportionately large suppressing effect on image contrast, that barriers must be laid in this plane too, to prevent its transmission. This arrangement, with two grids laid one

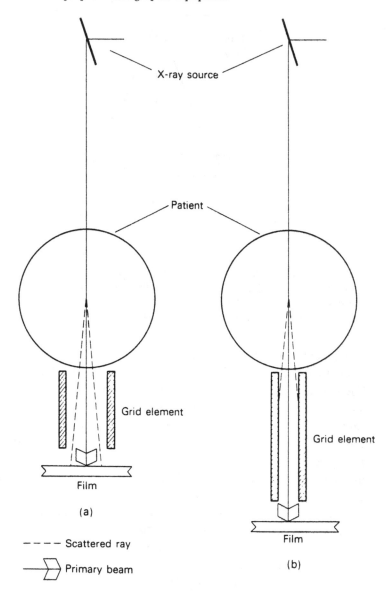

X-ray source

Patient

Grid element

Grid element

Film

(a)

– – – – Scattered ray

Primary beam

Film

(b)

**Fig. 5.6** The effect of grid ratio on scatter absorption. Oblique scatter at a narrow angular deviation from the primary ray penetrates a low ratio grid (a) but fails to get through the narrower interspace of a high ratio grid (b).

on top of the other, their lines mutually at right angles, forms what is known as a **crossed** or **cross-hatch** grid.

### Grid ratio
The efficiency with which a grid will absorb scattered radiation depends on the depth and narrowness of the radiolucent spaces or channels laid in its

path. If there is an oblique misalignment between scatter and a radiolucent channel, the scatter will strike and tend to be absorbed by the lead strip forming the channel's wall – if the channel is deep enough. This feature of a grid, determining how effectively a grid prevents transmission of scatter, is measured as the ratio between the *height* or *depth* of its radiolucent spaces, and their width. In practice, this ratio may be as low as 5:1 or as high as 16:1. The matching of a grid to its clinical use, in the matter of grid ratio, is not so much in the quantity of scatter produced as in its mean direction. The more *forward* the scatter, the greater the need for a high ratio. Thus, the 16:1 grid will principally find its application in techniques employing X-rays produced with a high tube kilovoltage.

### Grid factor

From the description of a grid given so far, it could be imagined that the best types of grid to use are high ratio grids, in cross-hatch formation. This strategy would cut scatter transmission to an absolute minimum! Unfortunately, it would also have a maximum effect in absorbing primary radiation, the consequence of which would be to raise the dose to the patient to a maximum value and lengthen the exposure time, with a consequently increased risk of movement unsharpness on the image.

Whenever a grid is used, these major disadvantages must be held in mind by radiographers.

The term **grid factor** is employed to indicate the multiple which needs to be applied to an exposure (the mAs) when a change in technique involves introducing the use of a grid. If the production of a radiograph without a grid requires $x$ mAs, while production of an identical image with a grid requires $6x$ mAs, the grid is said to have a factor of 6. In such a case, a decision must be made as to whether this six-fold increase in exposure – especially with regard to the patient's safety – is justified by the improvement in image contrast and enhancement of diagnostic value which the grid will bring. In practice, the need to make such decisions may be infrequent, involving only borderline cases.

### Grid line density

Used in a stationary position, a grid will tend to cast onto the image the pattern of its opaque strips as a series of fine, parallel, unexposed (clear) lines. The severity of this effect and its image break-up effect will be less in proportion to the fineness of the line density (lines per cm width across the grid).

Grids are now available which have a line density which is so fine that the naked eye cannot readily identify its pattern. Such grids tend to be very expensive, however, and the more usual, conventional method of eliminating grid lines from an image is by causing the grid to move transversely during an exposure. This movement blurs the grid line images beyond recognition. Movement still allows a grid to fulfil its scatter removing role, and has no effect on primary beam transmission.

### Grid movement

In order to be moved accurately and in a controlled manner, a grid has to be mounted in a frame, parallel to the imaging plane (film) and some form of movement mechanism has to be attached. This assembly is usually referred to as a **bucky** or a potter-bucky, after the names of its inventors.

A bucky grid is normally square (as opposed to the oblong shape of a stationary grid) to maintain coverage of all film sizes, despite its sideways excursion; the line density may be relatively coarse, since its super-imposition on images is prevented by movement.

Buckys are installed as integral parts of larger items of equipment: couches, vertical stands and fluoroscopic units. They usually incorporate cassette trays, and the whole assembly may be mounted on rails, so that its position can be moved and adjusted to relate to the anatomical region which is being radiographed. In a **pedestal** assembly, as with a floating-top table, grid location is fixed: the patient is moved, not the film.

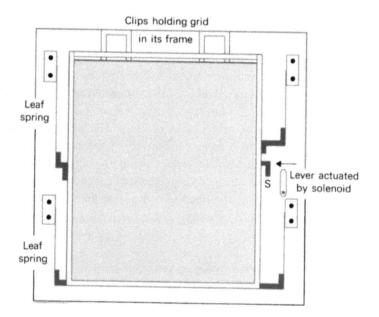

**Fig. 5.7** An oscillating bucky mechanism. The initial impulse at S sets the grid off, and its motion is maintained by the elastic action of the springs.

In modern equipment, bucky grid movement tends to be a simple, to-and-fro, sideways oscillation. In order to eliminate the risk of a stationary exposure, it is arranged for movement to begin before the start of an exposure; and initial movement must be fast, to maximize the blurring effect. The grid is mounted in a frame supported along its lateral borders by springs, against which the frame can bounce, to reverse its direction of travel. An initial thrust from an electromagnetic device, just before the exposure begins, sets the grid off in motion. After that, the grid's own momentum and the elastic effect of the springs are sufficient to maintain a pendulum like rhythmic movement. Naturally, this slows eventually to a halt but, under normal circumstances, not before the exposure has ended.

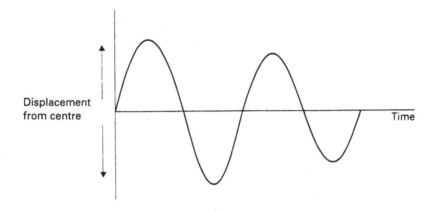

**Fig. 5.8** Graphical representation of the movement of an oscillating grid.

Despite its advantages, the routine use of grid movement has been questioned. It is argued that the bucky framework assembly increases the separation between patient and film to the detriment of the image's geometric unsharpness; that the movement mechanism (despite its reliability) represents yet another component which can fail and require repairing. There is a risk of a stationary exposure effect if a pulsating X-ray beam happens to synchronize with the grid's line spacing and speed (a stroboscopic effect) or during the motionless, neutral reverse points of its oscillation cycle. It may also be pointed out that, due to its displacement from the midline, for most of its travel X-ray beam and grid are mutually offcentred, with accompanying increased absorption of primary radiation.

These points need to be demonstrated in practice, however, and students will find that substitution of a fine line stationary grid, for a bucky, is a design feature of some equipment but not all. In situations where a cassette tray is required, the inclusion of a moving grid is still routine.

## 5.4 Follow-up practical

(1) The improvement in image contrast which collimation can produce is best appreciated by a *before and after* experiment. An anatomical phantom of a body part which is known to be responsible for a measurable amount of scatter – the abdomen, for example – should be used.

An initial radiograph without significant collimation is followed by a second for which the beam is collimated, say, to include only the vertebral column or an individual vertebra. The observable change in contrast should illustrate the advantage to the image, quite apart from the obvious reduction in radiation hazard.

(2) The test to measure coincidence of light and X-ray beams from an LBD should be performed. A deviation of 1% or less (e.g. 1 cm at a focus–film distance of 1 m) is considered to be tolerable.

Since the purpose of the test is to achieve confirmation that both light and X-rays are accurately aligned, the outcome may be unremarkable. It is useful, however, to consider the consequences of an undiscovered error – in terms, particularly, of its significance for patients.

(3) Students are recommended to survey the grids used in their own clinical placement areas. Grid sizes will vary, to match different sizes of films and cassettes, but other features need to be studied: these can be found printed or lightly embossed on the grids themselves. Are the grids that are used in the placement department parallel or focused; at what distances are they focused; what are their ratios; what are their line densities and what are their routine uses?

These enquiries may also include discovering differences in grid materials. The near zero absorption claimed for carbon fibre when used as an interspace material maximizes transmission of primary radiation. It also, however, allows scatter to pass easily through the interspaces. How, in practice, does this compare with the performance of an *all metal* grid which incorporates aluminium as its interspace material, which reduces transmission of scatter but also absorbs some primary radiation?

(4) The contrast improving properties of a grid may be demonstrated by experimental radiography of an anatomical phantom (a) without and (b) with a grid. These test exposures may also include investigation of the effects of the different types of grid identified in (3), above. As a result of these, some measurement can be made of grid factor and, possibly, some conclusions drawn about the particular suitability of one type of grid (or another) for a given radiographic examination.

(5) The misuse of a grid – beam angulation across instead of along the spaces, use at incorrect focus distances, offcentring and even use upside

down – can all be investigated, to reinforce appreciation of the need to align X-ray beam and grid correctly.

**(6)** Misuse of grids can sometimes be less technical but equally significant: they can be subjected to pressures and forces which they are physically unable to stand. Two points arise: how are grids normally protected against mishandling? And how can grid damage become apparent (as an artefact) on a radiographic image?

**(7)** Do the light-beam diaphragms also incorporate *dose × area product* devices? These are radiolucent ionization chambers connected to display and recording units. They do not interfere with the functioning of LBDs but may influence the care with which they are used. Each exposure produces a reading indicative of the quantity of radiation transmitted through the diaphragm aperture. Investigate the significance of these readings.

# Chapter 6
# Radiographic Couches, Stands and Tube Supports

## 6.1 X-ray tube supports

An X-ray tube typically weighs 25 kg or more. The need for a strong support to bear this weight is fundamental. There are other requirements, however, of practical importance:

(1) *The support must be accurately counterbalanced.* An equivalent weight or a counteracting spring must exert an upward force on the X-ray tube and its accessories (LBD, etc.) to match the gravitational force which seeks to bring it down. By this arrangement, the physical safety of both radiographer and patient is made more secure.

(2) *A range of free movements must be available.* Still supported, it must be possible to move the tube into different positions, so that the X-ray beam may be directed along horizontal, vertical and intermediate planes, and centred to a range of locations. This freedom allows the radiographer to perform the required range of standard and modified radiographic techniques.

(3) *The tube's position, in relation to all relevant planes and points, must be clearly measurable.* Distances include those from the tube's focal spot to reference planes such as the couch top, and the film/cassette plane within the couch, chest stand or vertical bucky.

While the LBD indicates beam centring to open areas such as a cassette placed on the couch top, calibrated reference scales and a positive centre lock device are needed to show when the tube is aligned to films and focused grids concealed within couch or vertical bucky.

Angles of tube rotation, both longitudinal and transverse, must be measurable to allow accuracy of radiographic techniques.

(4) *Immobilization locks need to be incorporated in the support.* When accurately placed in its required position, it must be possible for the tube to be immobilized quickly and securely.

(5) *Assisted drive mechanisms may be provided.* Electric motors which drive the tube support along and across the room and which adjust the

tube's height can reduce the physical stresses experienced by radiographers.

**(6)** *It may be necessary for a tomographic attachment to be fitted to the tube support.*

### Floor-mounted columns

The oldest design of tube support is a simple column, mounted on a wheeled base. This runs along a floor-mounted track, fixed parallel to the longitudinal axis of the couch, so that the tube can quite easily be moved from above the head to the foot of a recumbent patient, while remaining centred to the grid and film.

Increased stability may be given by an extended attachment to a ceiling track, aligned above the floor track. The column is frequently in the form of a hollow steel cylinder, around which is a strong, moveable sleeve or collar to which is fixed a cross-arm on which the X-ray tube is mounted. The tube's weight is carried by a steel cable which runs upwards, over a pulley and then down within the column where it is attached to a counterweight.

All movements can be locked, usually by quickly applied and released electromagnetic devices.

As well as holding the tube, the column has associated support arms, usually suspended from the ceiling track, which keep the tube supply cables out of harm's way – avoiding both damage and inconvenience.

A floor-mounted column offers the simplicity of construction and installation – for which reasons, it may still be seen in X-ray rooms – but it can form an obstacle for persons crossing the floor and its track can become an unhygienic trap for dust and dirt. Its main shortcoming, however, lies in the restriction of its transverse, horizontal movement. It is easily available for use with the couch and an aligned chest stand or vertical bucky, but offers little scope for performing techniques to examine patients on trolleys or in wheelchairs, elsewhere within the room.

### Ceiling-mounted tube supports

Ceiling-mounted tube supports – the most common, standard type – date from the time when X-ray departments began to occupy purpose-built accommodation, with strong ceilings! The tube is mounted on a telescopic column which projects down from a strong supporting carriage. The carriage is mounted on a set of rails which allow movement *across* the room and which are themselves mounted to travel at 90°, *along* the room. In this way, a large, rectangular area can be covered by the X-ray tube, well beyond the confines of the couch. Advantages, therefore, lie principally in wide-ranging positioning opportunities throughout the room, both for use and storage.

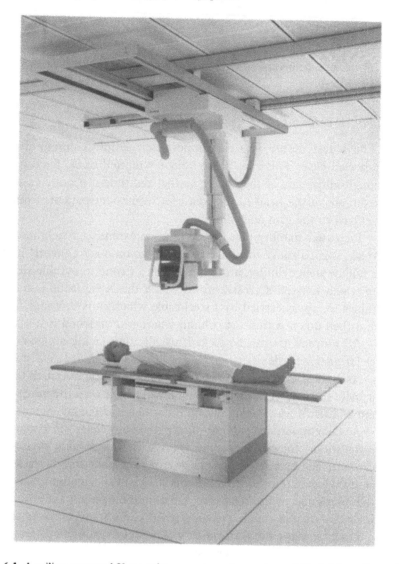

**Fig. 6.1** A ceiling-mounted X-ray tube support carriage and a variable height radiographic couch. The X-ray tube may be centred to the film in the bucky unit but it is also free to be used for radiographing patients, for example on trolleys or in wheelchairs, anywhere within the extent of its large, rectangular area. (*By courtesy of Siemens plc.*)

Counterbalancing, distance indicators and motorized, assisted movement mechanisms are all incorporated within the supporting carriage.

## 6.2 Radiographic couches

Radiographic couches or tables meet most or all of the following criteria:

(1) Strongly constructed to bear the weight of a heavy patient in safety.
(2) Incorporating a grid and cassette tray, usually as a bucky assembly, which can be aligned to any part of the patient's body, for convenient and easy radiographic positioning.
(3) Incorporating radiation protection screens against scattered radiation emerging from the exposed cassette and from other structures lying below the couch top, in the path of the primary beam.
(4) Electrically safe, with earthing of all exposed metallic parts.
(5) The couch top must be:
   (a) Long enough and wide enough to accommodate the largest of patients, in safety.
   (b) At a height which allows both safe access for a patient and comfortable working (not causing a risk of back strain, for instance) for the radiographer.
   (c) Radiolucent, to allow free transmission of the primary beam.
   (d) Made of materials which are not easily scratched: both to allow hygiene to be maintained and to prevent the risk that damage or ingrained foreign matter may cause artefacts to appear on radiographs.
   (e) Marked in some way – typically by a prominent central line – (unless it is 'floating') to allow the X-ray beam to be centred accurately from outside to the grid and film inside.
   (f) Bordered along its sides by rails of some kind, to which accessories can be fitted.
(6) Additionally, there may be advantages (depending on its location) in the couch having the facility of being tilted from a horizontal to a vertical position.

### Couch top materials

The combination of strength, radiolucency and resistance to damage, is found in a range of mineral/plastic compounds, but the most efficient performance is found in carbon fibre.

### Alignment of the patient to the film

The grid/cassette assembly comprises a grid – either stationary or with a movement mechanism (bucky) – close below the undersurface of the couch top, with a cassette tray beneath. If fitted, autotimer chambers may lie between the grid and the film. The cassette tray has a pair of reciprocating clamps which guide cassettes into a central position, underneath the midline of the couch. As an elaboration of this arrangement, sensors may be fitted to detect cassette size. These feed back a signal to the collimator, to ensure that the primary field cannot exceed the film's area, as a radiation protection precaution. The whole assembly has a wheeled mounting on longitudinal rails, along which it can move, from one end of the couch to the other, to cover most of the length of a recumbent patient. A lock allows it to be immobilized in position, as required, in relation to the anatomical area being examined.

### Fixed couches

The simplest of couches is fixed to the floor on legs and has an immovable top. The patient has to be pulled or otherwise manoeuvred into position, as required by the radiographer, for alignment with the X-ray beam, grid and film. While this design may be cheap and offer the most compact arrangement within a restricted space, it is awkward, if not hazardous, for radiographers and patients alike.

### Moving tops

An improvement in ease of use is to be found in couches which have a moving top. The basic movement is simply in a longitudinal direction, driven by an electric motor, with low gear, gentle control. It allows even the tallest patient to be accommodated by the film's area, without having to be pulled by the radiographer along the couch. If the couch can also be tilted, the moving top facility allows an erect patient to be raised and lowered for convenience when radiographs are taken with a horizontal beam.

Transverse as well as longitudinal movement is offered by the **floating top** couch. This is a stage more complicated than a simple moving top: two sets of horizontal support frames, one above the other, allow the top to be moved both across and along a stationary central pedestal which houses the grid/cassette assembly, to which the X-ray beam is centred. (This two-directional movement copies the flexibility which a ceiling-mounted tube support offers.)

The extra movement is possible at the expense of a larger gap between the film plane below and the couch top above. This may be criticized as a source of increasing geometric unsharpness – in response to which some manufacturers produce a **dished** couch top, i.e. one with a recessed, broad channel along its length. This can comfortably accommodate most recumbent patients but can pose problems for couch-top techniques with a horizontal beam.

The important advantage of a floating top couch, however, is its ease of operation when the patient is being positioned. Movements are free-running, either hand-controlled or servo-assisted by electric motors, and locks are easily applied, either by hand or pedal controls. As a result,

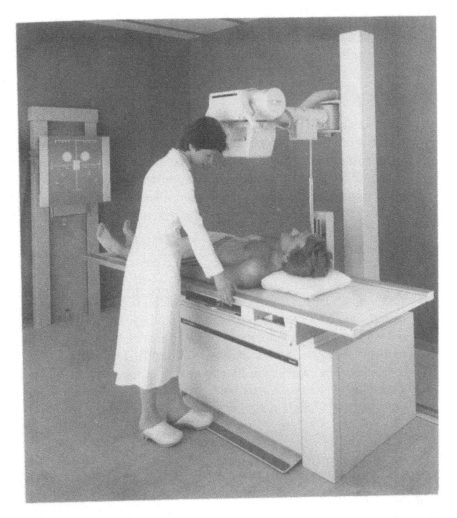

**Fig. 6.2** An X-ray tube on a floor-mounted column, coupled with a floating top radiographic couch. The tube is also aligned to a vertical bucky, for horizontal beam techniques. A tomographic attachment is seen fitted, linking tube and couch. The table top locks are released and applied by a foot-operated bar. (*By courtesy of Philips Medical Systems.*)

positioning can be quick and effortless – a particular advantage when the patient has suffered trauma or when the examination involves several parts of the body.

### Tilting couches

Tilting couches are normally associated with fluoroscopic rather than radiographic use. They require a very strong, stable, floor mounting, off-centred towards the end of the couch which is normally lowered during tilting. The strength of this mount can be appreciated when it is realized that it fulfils the function of the legs on a fixed couch. As with the couch top, motorized movement must be gentle, low geared and instantly controllable by the operator. For convenience, there may be two speeds.

### Variability of height

The problem of finding a couch height which is convenient and accessible both for the radiographer bending down, and for patients climbing up or transferring from a trolley, is only solved successfully by a variable height couch. A central, strong telescoping support is motor-driven, usually with pedal controls, up or down to the required level. Inclusion of a floating top completes the convenience and makes this design popular with all who use it.

### Accessories

The rails which run along the longitudinal borders of the couch top have grooves into which a range of accessories can be fitted, to assist radiographer and patient. The compression (displacement) and immobilization band is probably the commonest accessory. Support items – hand grips, shoulder rests, footsteps, supporting harnesses and bands – are usually associated with tilting couches. Cassette holders (for horizontal beam techniques) and support stands for other equipment may also be used.

## 6.3 Chest stands and vertical buckys

### Chest stand

This is simply a holder for a vertically positioned cassette, supported on either a floor mounted column or a wall mounted frame. Vertical adjustment is provided to match patients' varying heights.

### Vertical bucky

This has most of the features of a radiographic couch top:

(1) A radiolucent front surface, marked to show the midline and the locations of autotimer chambers. It may have a notch in its upper border, to form a chin rest for patients having their chests radiographed (postero-anterior projection).
(2) A grid, either moving or stationary, with its lines vertical, to suit the beam angulations most commonly required by radiographic techniques. It may also be possible for the cassette/grid assembly to be rotated – still

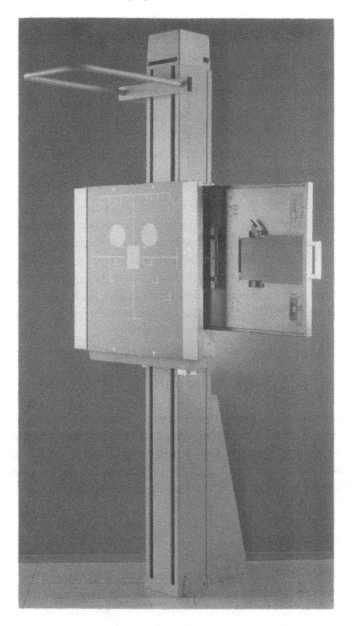

**Fig. 6.3** A vertical bucky unit. The floor mounted column is equipped with a handrail accessory for lateral chest radiography. Markings on the front indicate centring axes, film sizes and the locations of the autotimer ionization chambers. The cassette tray is in an open position, showing the cassette holding devices. (*By courtesy of Philips Medical Systems.*)

in a vertical plane – through 90°, so that the grid lines are horizontal.
(3) A cassette tray, possibly with extra guides to centring, to combat the downward slide of a cassette against its vertical surface.
(4) Side rails or other provisions for fitment of accessories, including a chest-stand cassette support.

A vertical bucky is either wall mounted or on a stout, floor mounted column (or twin columns) with counterbalanced movement through a wide range of heights. Its applications therefore extend beyond the chest to other anatomical areas.

Angulation may be possible from its normally vertical position into a horizontal plane. It can then be used as a supplementary, variable height couch for certain examinations and as a grid/cassette unit in conjunction with a radiolucent-top trolley for trauma patients.

It is common for fixed chest stands (some are moveable) and vertical buckys to be aligned to the central axis of the room's radiographic couch. The calibrated scales and the locking device which indicate tube centring to the couch then also guide the radiographer when performing techniques with a vertical film in the stand or bucky.

## 6.4 Modern basic radiographic units

Equipment is becoming more common, in which tube mount and couch are integrated. Versatility of movement allows all the principal radiographic procedures to be performed with the minimum of physical effort on the radiographer's part. This allows examinations to be carried out more efficiently and accurately than when components are separate.

## 6.5 Follow-up practical

Carefully examine examples of these common items of equipment within clinical departments. Carry out a comparison between two units which serve similar purposes – two couches, two tube supports – which are of different design. Which is found easier by radiographers – and by patients? What key points account for these preferences – accuracy, ease-of-use, reliability?

# Part Four
# Fluoroscopic Equipment

Radiographic images are limited:

(1) Only stationary objects are shown; there is no demonstration of movement. In fact, since movement causes image unsharpness, it is deliberately excluded.

(2) Radiographic techniques employ positioning procedures which, although performed with skill, are essentially *blind*, being based on informed expectation rather than individual certainty. In most instances, routine positioning is sufficient to yield a successful diagnosis but there are exceptions, where unpredictable anatomical variations or pathological abnormalities are revealed.

(3) Radiographic images become visible only after a delay, while some form of processing takes place.

Contrasting with these limitations, there are instances where a reliable radiological diagnosis depends on:

(1) Demonstration of movement, for example as evidence of function: when the patient's body needs to be *watched* rather than simply *seen*.

(2) Positioning undertaken with a precision requiring knowledge of the patient's particular, individual characteristics.

(3) Immediate imaging, as rapid feedback to the operator; during surgery, for example, or other interventional procedures.

In situations such as these, where images need to be dynamic, immediate or matched to some individual structural feature, the preferred procedure is fluoroscopy, rather than radiography. Chapter 7 describes equipment designed for these purposes.

# Chapter 7
# Fluoroscopic Equipment

## 7.1 Introduction

In a fluoroscopic set-up, the transmitted X-ray beam emerging from the patient is incident on the sensitive input area of an **image intensifier**, positioned where the film would be in a radiographic procedure.

Initially (as with intensifying screens in a cassette) the incident X-ray pattern is converted into a visible light image. This is then immediately converted into an electron emission pattern. Then, energy is added to produce a greatly intensified, dynamic, *real time* image which is scanned by a television camera and displayed on a monitor screen.

Thus, under *fluoroscopic control*, there is immediate display of the patient's body. Motion of organs or the flow of contrast media can be watched, and fine adjustments can be made to the patient's position or the position of an inserted instrument such as a catheter, to secure an exact diagnostic image.

It may be appropriate to mention terminology at this juncture. Fluoroscopy originated as a technique in which images from the transmitted X-ray beam were formed on a primitive fluoroscopic screen. For simplicity, this procedure was known as **screening** (possibly to distinguish it from **filming**). For colloquial use within an imaging department, the term screening may well survive for ever; but students need to recognize – and take care to avoid – an ambiguity. Increasing emphasis on preventive medicine has brought the term screening into prominence, to mean an investigation conducted on a specific population, in search of (to eliminate or confirm) a specific disease or condition. This general usage impinges on radiography. For example, while it may involve the use of X-rays, *breast screening* has no connection at all with fluoroscopy.

The term fluoroscopy is sometimes avoided on the grounds of awkwardness. It forms no convenient verb – 'I'm going to fluoroscope this patient' (?) – and many students find the word difficult to spell. Nevertheless, particularly when discussing this procedure outside the confines of an imaging department, proper reference to *fluoroscopy* and *fluoroscopic equipment* should be observed.

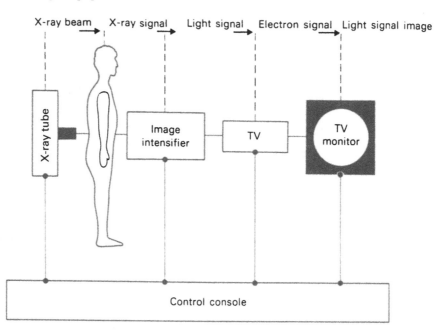

X-ray beam   X-ray signal   Light signal   Electron signal   Light signal image

**Fig. 7.1** Summary of the signal conversion stages during fluoroscopy. The *radiation image* originally created by the X-ray beam is converted into a visible image within the image intensifier and then immediately converted into an *electron image*. This is intensified and reconverted to a visible light image (output) which is scanned by a television camera, and so converted into an electronic video signal. The video signal is fed to a television monitor, where it is redisplayed as a visible image, and/or digitized for manipulation, prior to being recorded as a hard copy.

## X-ray tube alignment to the image intensifier

Radiographic and fluoroscopic equipment differ in the way that the X-ray tube is mounted. Tubes used for radiography commonly have unrestricted movement. The X-ray beam can be centred to films positioned in bucky equipment (vertical or horizontal), on a couch top, trolley or elsewhere. This lack of restriction is required by the freedom and convenience of the film cassette, usable in a wide variety of situations, to cover any required anatomical area. This freedom can create problems, however: radiation field alignment and collimation to the film area can be complicated by angulations and varying distances.

In contrast to the ease of positioning a cassette, an image intensifier is a relatively awkward piece of equipment: it is bulky, heavy and delicate. A benefit of this awkwardness is a limitation on the fluoroscopic tube's need for freedom: since it can only be used when centred to its image intensifier, provision for beam centring and collimation is simplified. It is always the case, therefore, that a fluoroscopic X-ray tube is rigidly linked to an image intensifier. Accurate X-ray beam centring is thus achieved, as are a maximum field size and shape, matched exactly to the image intensifier input area.

## 7.2 Types of fluoroscopic equipment

The principle of having the X-ray tube rigidly linked and permanently centred to an imaging device is becoming familiar in radiography, through the introduction of isocentric equipment. A similar and fairly familiar unit, the mobile image intensifier, provides a simple illustration of the fluoroscopic principle. X-ray tube and image intensifier are mounted at opposing points of a **C-arm**. The anatomical part to be examined is placed within the X-ray beam passing from tube to intensifier. If the object lies at the central point (isocentre) about which both tube and intensifier rotate, movement of the assembly can produce any chosen image (projection) without need to move the patient. This satisfies the desirable principle of fitting the equipment to the patient, rather than the opposite: requiring patients to be manoeuvred in relation to a rigidly predetermined beam. C-arm and U-arm mountings allow operators to perform procedures, including complex, interventional work, with the facility of X-ray beam angulations refined to any direction, in any plane – all without requiring the patient to be moved from a basic position.

Fluoroscopic equipment of an earlier and still familiar design provides no such convenience for the patient. The conventional fluoroscopic couch incorporates an X-ray tube rigidly linked to an image intensifier, but with an X-ray beam limited to being directed at right angles to the couch top. The couch, similar in most respects to a tilting radiographic couch, is fitted with an assembly which supports the intensifier and its aligned X-ray tube, plus all the operating controls.

## 7.3 Conventional fluoroscopic couches

A fluoroscopic couch is basically a tilting radiographic couch, capable of a full 90° forward movement and either limited reverse tilting (typically 30°) or a full reverse 90°. Standard accessories are fitted to the couch top: a footrest for the patient when tilting towards an erect position, and other supports: hand grips, shoulder supports and other aids. The fixed direction of the X-ray beam means that the patient has to turn or be turned into position, if a comprehensive examination (a barium enema, for example) is to be conducted. Some manufacturers offer a rotating cradle as an optional extra. This goes some way towards making the equipment less demanding on the patient, particularly the disabled and the very young. Once installed in the cradle and restrained with safety straps, patients can be rotated without effort on their part.

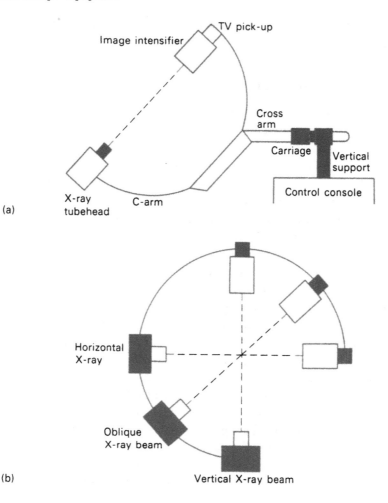

**Fig. 7.2** Principle of an isocentric, C-arm image intensifier (mobile). (a) Tube and intensifier are exactly aligned and rigidly coupled. Maximum X-ray field cannot exceed the area of the intensifier's input screen. (b) Once the unit is positioned with the anatomical subject at the centre of rotation, any angulation (projection) can be achieved, within the limitations of the rotational planes available.

   The couch offers a provision for conducting fluoroscopy, in that an X-ray tube and image intensifier are permanently attached; the patient lying on or standing in front of the couch top is examined by the X-ray beam passing from the tube to the intensifier. Attached to the intensifier is a television camera which scans the intensified image and displays it on a monitor screen adjacent to, but separate from, the couch. In addition to the television camera, there may be a fluorographic camera – although such cameras are now disappearing from use, being replaced with more efficient and versatile digital imaging systems.

There are two basic equipment designs. The older of the two incorporates an X-ray tube under the couch, built into a framework which links it to a moveable assembly, termed an **explorator**. This bears the image intensifier and its associated camera equipment. The newer design has the image intensifier under the couch, while the X-ray tube is above.

## The under-couch tube design

The over-couch explorator incorporates an image intensifier, accurately centred and aligned to the X-ray beam from the under-couch tube. The explorator is counterbalanced so that it is virtually *weightless* for safe and easy movement up and down (along) or from side to side across the patient's body. Such movement is necessary because the imaging field is naturally restricted. Motor drive assistance is normally provided, to reduce the effort required by the operator.

Recording of permanent images on film (*hard copy*) may be via a digital system or, on older equipment, via a fluorographic camera which is used to

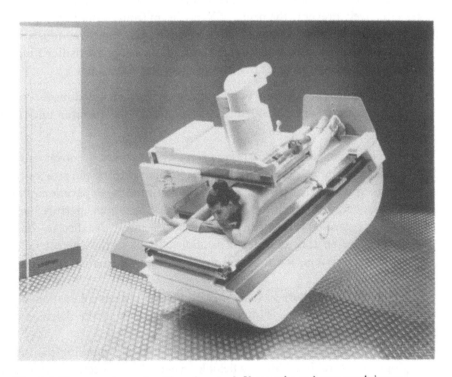

**Fig. 7.3** Fluoroscopic couch with under-couch X-ray tube and over-couch image intensifier. The couch, fitted with a footrest, is shown with an adverse, *head down* tilt from its horizontal position. The controls can be seen on the explorator which links the supported image intensifier to the X-ray tube (out of sight, below the couch top). (*By courtesy of Siemens plc.*)

photograph selected images from the intensifier onto miniature (100 mm) film. If the equipment is even older, the explorator may also offer the facility of exposing X-ray films in full-size cassettes. These are loaded into a moveable frame at the side of the intensifier which, on the 'spot film' exposure command, is driven across to a position in front of the intensifier input, where a radiographic exposure is given. In conjunction with protective metal masks on the explorator surface nearest the patient, a cassette can be given a series of small field exposures. In this way, for both speed and economy, a single film can record up to six images.

A device for applying localized compression to the patient's abdomen can be fitted to the front of the explorator and a fine-line or moving grid can be fitted in front of the cassette plane.

All the controls for explorator movement and locking, couch tilt, beam collimation and exposure are mounted on the explorator for convenient use by the operator.

### Radiation protection

The image intensifier is surrounded by a lead-lined housing which effectively prevents the primary X-ray beam from presenting a hazard to its operator. The boundaries of the beam emitted by the X-ray tube are limited so that the radiation field does not exceed the image intensifier's input area. This precaution ensures that the primary beam does not

(1) irradiate the patient's body outside the area included on the image; or
(2) present a direct hazard to the equipment's operator and to other personnel in attendance.

This limitation is complicated by the permitted movement of the explorator towards and away from the patient (for the purpose of reducing geometric unsharpness and magnification, or for the application of localized tissue compression). If the beam collimator (maximum aperture) were to be fixed to cover the intensifier's input at its closest distance to the tube, it would exceed this at wider separations. If set to the correct field at the widest separation, it would fail to show the full imaging area at a shorter distance.

Accordingly, there is an automatic linkage between collimation and tube–intensifier separation. This ensures safety, whatever the distance between the tube and the intensifier.

The explorator incorporates lead protection surrounding the intensifier input aperture. In addition, a flexible lead-rubber protective apron or skirt is attached around the margin of the explorator, to absorb scattered radiation. The gap beneath the couch top which normally allows access to a bucky assembly (for insertion and removal of a cassette) may be closed by a protective flap during fluoroscopy, as an extra measure for absorbing scatter.

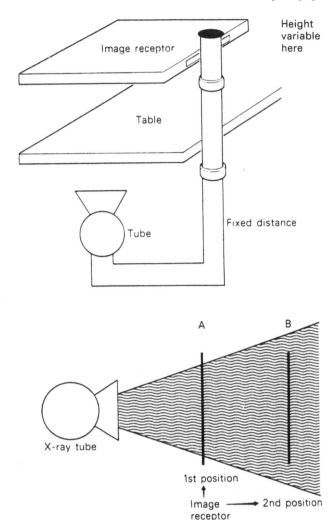

**Fig. 7.4** Limitation of the primary X-ray field from an under-couch X-ray tube, in a fluoroscopic unit. (a) The tube is fitted within a carriage which keeps it at a fixed distance from the table top. The image intensifier (within the explorator), however, can be moved in towards and out, away from the table top. (b) Automatic adjustment of the collimators ensures that the X-ray field never exceeds the area of the image intensifier input. Movement of the explorator away from the table top, from A to B, requires the automatic device to collimate the beam more narrowly, otherwise exposure outside the margins of the image intensifier input screen will occur, with consequently increased hazards to the patient and the operator.

All fluoroscopic equipment includes an **integrating timer**. This is a device which measures and adds together the separate time bursts when the X-ray tube is energized. Usual practice is for this total time to be allowed to accumulate up to, but not beyond, a prespecified safety limit. It is therefore incumbent on the operator to be extremely careful, exposing the patient only when necessary so that the examination is completed within the time allowed.

## The over-couch tube design

The under-couch tube design originated at a time when the operator viewed a direct fluoroscopic screen, i.e. before the introduction of image intensification. This type of equipment has the advantage of allowing the operator and other attending personnel to be close to the patient: for easy communication and reassurance and, except when the tube is energized, for handling accessory equipment and palpation.

The alternative equipment configuration, with the X-ray tube above the couch top and the image intensifier below, offers the advantage of allowing a greater distance between the tube and both the patient and intensifier. This

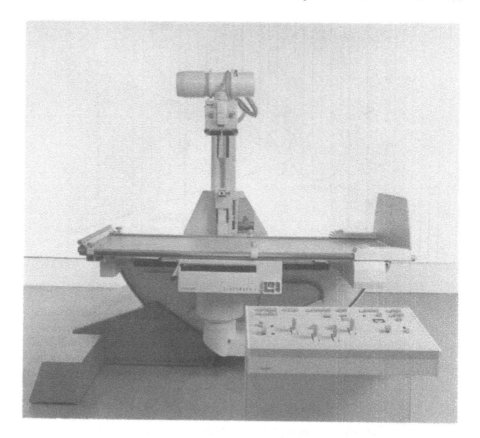

**Fig. 7.5** Remote-control fluoroscopic couch with over-couch X-ray tube and under-couch image intensifier. The remote console is shown with its array of controls. The operator sits behind a lead glass screen which affords a full view of the patient on the couch. (*By courtesy of Siemens plc.*)

tends to improve image quality by reducing geometric unsharpness and it can reduce the radiation skin dose to the patient. It also, however, effectively excludes the patient management techniques used with under-couch tube equipment: radiation hazards to the operator – principally from scatter but also conceivably from the primary beam – would be prohibitively high.

Accordingly, this type of equipment was designed for remote-control operation. The operator sits at a distance, behind a transparent protective barrier, at a console, operating the equipment's controls (couch tilt, couch top movement, application of compression and exposure) while viewing the monitor screen. Communication with the patient is conducted via some form of amplified two-way system. The patient's relatively open situation is considered to be less threatening than when restricted by the closeness of an explorator, although, to offset this, the patient may suffer from a sense of isolation.

The shortcomings of remote-control fluoroscopic equipment arise from the separation between staff and patient. They include the need to have a contingency procedure for quickly attending patients who require emergency help – a fact which may indicate the unsuitability of this type of equipment for certain patients.

The couch may have a standard bucky facility to enable it to be used for radiography when not required for fluoroscopy. If so, the bucky assembly is automatically moved away into a parked location, clear of the image intensifier, when fluoroscopy is conducted, returning to a central position beneath the couch top when radiographic use is selected. Judicious, controlled use of the equipment's fluoroscopic facility can be a useful adjunct to its radiographic use, if employed to provide a brief positioning check prior to exposure, in selected cases where some doubt may exist about the object's normality. This facility is best employed in conjunction with a fluoroscopic 'memory' spot exposure system.

### Radiation protection

Since the equipment is designed to provide full protection for personnel, attention is focused fully on reducing hazards to the patient. The dose-reducing effect of the greater tube–patient distance may be significant. The operator's vigilance with collimation and observation of the need to minimize the integrated (cumulative) exposure time are also paramount.

## 7.4 Mobile and specialized fluoroscopic units

A C-arm mobile image intensifier incorporates an X-ray tube permanently aligned to a small input (typically 15 cm) intensifier with its attached television camera. The unit, on its wheeled base, is positioned to enclose or

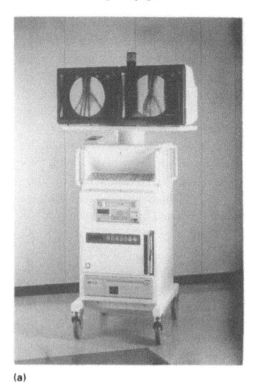
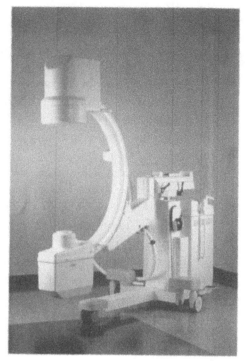

(a)                                        (b)

Fig. 7.6 A C-arm mobile image intensifier. (a) The dual-monitor unit, with its memory, recording and hard-copy facilities. (b) The C-arm tube/intensifier unit with integral X-ray generator. (*By courtesy of IGE Medical Systems.*)

surround the object which is being examined. The equipment is versatile, being capable of a range of movements, rotational and vertical. There is no patient support, however: a radiolucent trolley or table or other support is required.

An X-ray generator supplies energy to the X-ray tube, and a high tension supply is required for the image intensifier. The size and cost of the unit may be minimized by the incorporation of a stationary anode X-ray tube. In most situations, a satisfactory, intensified image can be produced while the required rate of X-ray emission can remain relatively low. The accompanying television monitor (commonly twin provision, in association with a memory, for simultaneous display of two projections) is on a trolley, connected via a cable from the television camera.

A higher rate of X-ray production is required when fluoroscopy is provided for specialized (e.g. cardiovascular) procedures in the imaging department. A rotating anode X-ray tube and a large field image intensifier are incorporated into a fully automated and versatile unit, in a U-arm or C-arm configuration. This may be ceiling mounted, to keep floor space free for the many other equipment units needed during such procedures. The

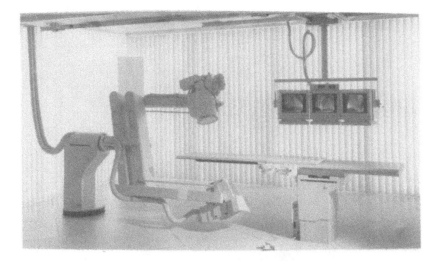

**Fig. 7.7** A floor mounted, U-arm fluoroscopic system. Complete versatility of angulation (projection) is offered by the combination of motor-driven movements, in all planes, while the patient lies on the independent, carbon-fibre couch top. (*By courtesy of Philips Medical Systems.*)

patient lies on a special radiolucent, extended table which may also be ceiling mounted. Refinements include computer memory recording of the optimum angulations established during the investigation, to allow quick, accurate reproduction of projections. The video signal, invariably digitized, can be fed to subtraction, enhancement and many other facilities.

## 7.5 The image intensifier

### Introduction

Image intensification is not confined to X-ray imaging; another application is night-time surveillance. These two improbably matched situations have something in common: an unsatisfactorily low level of lighting. This confirms that the essential purpose of an image intensifier is to convert a dim image into a bright one.

The dimness of a night-time landscape is familiar. The equivalent problem in X-ray imaging is probably less obvious. Before image intensification was introduced, fluoroscopy was performed with a simple fluoroscopic screen. Basically, this comprised a fluorescent layer sandwiched between a base support through which it was exposed, and a thick sheet of lead glass through which it was viewed. The average level of light emission from the screen was so low that it required the room to be in complete darkness. Under these inconvenient and potentially hazardous conditions,

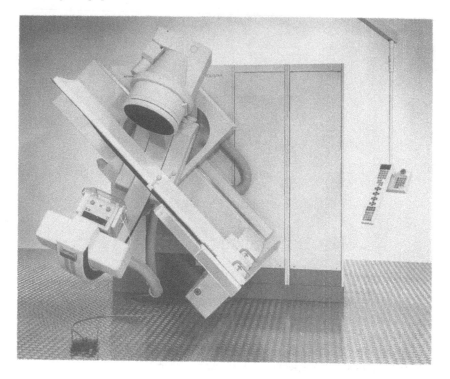

**Fig. 7.8** A C-arm fluoroscopic unit with tilting, integral examination table. The universal angulation provided by the C-arm allows any projection to be achieved, while the patient remains simply recumbent or leaning back against the couch top. The image intensifier may be positioned either above (in front of) or below (behind) the couch top. This arrangement offers a freedom which contrasts with the inherent restrictions of a conventional fluoroscopic couch. The television camera, which can be seen adjacent to the image intensifier, feeds a video signal to the digitized imaging equipment. (*By courtesy of Siemens plc.*)

the dim image was difficult to see. If strenuous efforts were made to interpret it, the examination tended to be overprolonged, quite often to the discomfort or distress of the patient.

A fluoroscopic screen could be made brighter only by increasing the intensity of the X-ray beam. This involved raising the tube current and possibly also the kilovoltage. Unavoidably, therefore, an accompanying rise occurred in the radiation dose rate to the patient.

## Construction and operation

The X-ray image intensifier is a large evacuated envelope, exposed at its front to receive the X-ray beam emerging from the patient, but otherwise encased by lead protection, to minimize X-ray leakage. Its metallic housing is lead lined around the sides and incorporates a small, lead glass aperture at the back, through which there is access to the output image. The envelope is cylindrical, made of glass or metal (titanium is widely used, combining strength with minimal X-ray absorption). The diameter of the circular input is normally within the range 15 to 30 cm; varying according to the clinical purpose of the intensifier. A larger diameter increases the viewable field size but it also increases the equipment's bulk and cost.

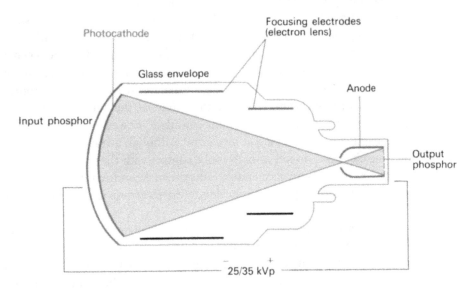

**Fig. 7.9** Principal features of an X-ray image intensifier tube. The shaded area shows the path of the electron beam, converging from its emission at the photocathode down to a point at the anode, before diverging to form a small, inverted image on the output phosphor.

The front of the envelope is convex, for optical reasons: to maintain a constant distance between every point on the input image and the eventual output image. Close within its surface is a layer of fluorescent material which serves the same purpose as in the former fluoroscopic screen: it converts X-rays into visible light. The phosphor normally now used for this **input screen** is sodium-activated caesium iodide. This material combines high X-ray absorption and energy conversion with a favourable crystal shape – like needles which, end-on to the screen surface, create high resolution.

The light image formed on this input phosphor cannot be viewed directly. If it could be, it would still be classified as relatively *dim*, with all the accompanying problems. Instead, the first stage of the intensification process begins. Closely applied to the input screen (though electrically insulated from it by a very thin layer of glass) is a layer which forms the intensifier's electrical cathode. This is made of compounds of caesium or antimony. Its function is to emit electrons when it receives energy. This energy is not required to be in the form of heat (as an X-ray tube filament, for example) but in the form of light. Its light-sensitive and electron-emitting properties give this structure the term **photocathode**.

The photocathode emits electrons from all points within its area at rates in proportion to the exciting light intensities – which are themselves proportional to the incident X-ray intensities. The emitted *electron image* thus accurately represents the original X-ray image.

At this stage, energy is given to the electrons. Like electrons crossing an X-ray tube, the electrons which form the image on the photocathode are given energy by a kilovoltage applied across the intensifier, between the photocathode and the anode. From their relatively large source, the electrons are focused by the electric fields emitted by surrounding electrodes, to form a converging beam, reducing to a point at the centre of the anode. Resemblance to an X-ray tube is not complete, however. The intensifier's anode has a circular opening at its centre. Although attracted by its electric field, the electrons do not actually make contact with the anode. Its function is therefore to act as an accelerator, rather than a conducting electrode. The potential difference applied to accelerate the electrons is in the range 25 to 35 kV.

With their momentum, the electrons pass through the anode where, now shielded from the focusing fields, they diverge before striking the final part of the insert, the **output phosphor** layer. The material used here is zinc cadmium sulphide, activated with silver. This has the purpose of (re)converting the electrons' energy into visible light. It should be stressed that the image is formed not by the electrons themselves but by their energy. The electrons leave the intensifier via a conducting path incorporated into the output layer.

The electron beam's cross-over, at the point where it enters the anode, causes the image to be inverted. This is of little consequence. What is important is that each point within the original image formed on the input phosphor layer is now accurately recreated on the visible image formed at the output.

It is technically possible for the output image to be viewed directly by the eye (although, in practice, this would be most unusual). If this were to occur, the image would be rated as *bright* – certainly in comparison with the original. This brightness gain, the intensification, occurs due to a combination of two effects. First, through the energy given to the electrons by the kilovoltage applied across the intensifier; and second, by the concentration of the image, from a diameter of between 15 and 30 cm, to a diameter of 3 to 4 cm.

Most intensifiers offer a dual-field or triple-field facility which enables a restricted central part of the input to have its image magnified up to the full size of the viewing area. This is achieved by altering the electrical field strength exerted by the focusing electrodes.

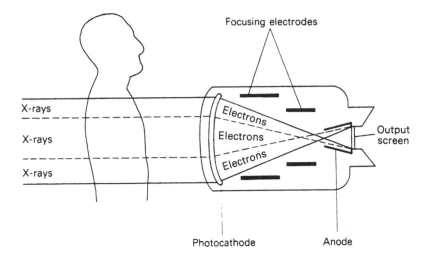

**Fig. 7.10** A dual-field image intensifier tube. The output (viewed screen) shows the whole of the area covered by the X-ray field. Selective use of its central part (shown by broken lines) can produce a magnified image for closer investigation of an area of particular interest.

The optical integrity of the intensifier is maintained by accurate alignment of the permanent structures, and accuracy and uniformity of the electric fields. Deviations from established values may cause effects on the image. Distortion can occur so that straight lines within the object can appear curved: inwards, to form a *barrel* effect; outwards, to form a *pincushion* effect. Image intensity can vary within the field area – typically fading around the perimeter, to form the *vignetting* effect. Deterioration of the phosphor layers causes loss of resolution, while focusing inaccuracies can introduce a loss of image definition.

### Image distribution and viewing

The intensified fluoroscopic image is invariably viewed via a closed-circuit television system. A television camera is therefore lined up to the image intensifier's output, to relay it to a monitor screen. Modern practice is for the video signal to be digitized and employed in a digital imaging system. If a camera is used (photofluorography or more simply fluorography), some provision must be made for allowing the output from the intensifier to be viewed simultaneously by both the television and the fluorographic camera. This is achieved by use of an image distributor (also sometimes known as a **beam splitter**).

The image from the intensifier passes to the television camera through a *tandem* system of optical lenses. This system can be interrupted, at a point where the light forms a parallel beam, by a special type of mirror which is set at an angle of 45° to the light beam's axis, so that it can both reflect and

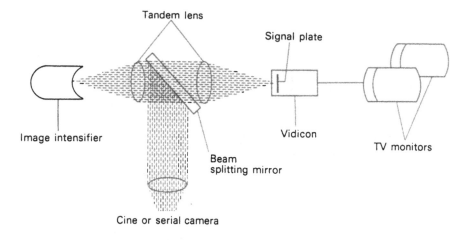

**Fig. 7.11** Use of a fluorographic camera. The light rays transmitted from the image intensifier ouptut to the television camera can be intercepted when a tandem lens coupling is employed: interception by a beam-splitting mirror both reflects (90%) and transmits (10%), allowing simultaneous use of both television and fluorographic cameras.

transmit. Because the television camera, in contrast to a fluorographic camera, can make electronic compensation for low light levels, the balance of distribution is typically 90% reflected to the fluorographic camera and 10% transmitted through to the television camera. Two fluorographic cameras may be used – a cine camera and a 105 mm *spot film* camera, for example – when there is a provision for the image distributor to be rotated, to reflect the intensifier's output to either one camera or the other.

Any optical system is subject to a loss of performance which may cause image deterioration. If the sole means of viewing the image intensifier's output is the television camera, and recording is via the electronic video signal, an alternative form of linkage may be used. This comprises a bundle of fine optical fibres which, point-by-point, link the intensifier output image to the television camera input. This system allows no interruption, however: no alternative image distribution is permitted.

## 7.6  Television cameras

The commonest type of television camera used in fluoroscopy systems is termed a **vidicon**. This is an evacuated glass tube, 2 to 3 cm in diameter and 15–20 cm long. The image from the intensifier is focused onto the camera's input, target end. This comprises three layers:

(1) Outermost is a glass **face plate**, continuous with the tube's envelope. It protects and supports the two layers which lie inside it.

(2) Coated onto the glass is a layer of zinc oxide, forming the **signal electrode**. This has two properties: it is an electrical conductor and it is transparent. The transparency allows the light image to pass through onto the next, innermost layer.

(3) This is a mosaic (an array of millions of tiny photoelectric cells) of antimony trisulphide, a material which is a **photoconductor**, that is its conductivity is affected by the presence of light energy. When illuminated, it conducts more freely than when it is dark.

At the opposite end of the camera tube is a composite structure, termed an electron *gun*. This comprises:

(1) A **filament**, heated to emit electrons;
(2) A **grid** which controls rate of electron flow, through to
(3) An **accelerating electrode**. This has an open centre through which pass the electrons as a very fine, narrow beam.

Across the camera, as a whole, is a potential difference of between 20 and 60 V.

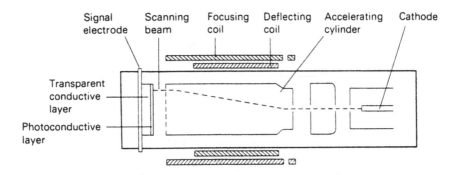

**Fig. 7.12** Simplified sectional diagram of a vidicon television camera tube.

After emerging from the gun, the electron beam comes under the influence of electric fields created by coils situated closely around (outside) the glass tube. These focus the electron beam onto the photoconductor layer and, by a combination of horizontal and vertical deflection, cause it to move through a **scanning** pattern cycle. The beam traces horizontal lines across the area, moving from the top to the bottom, rather like the eye reading this printed page of text. On reaching the bottom right-hand corner, the beam flies back diagonally to the top left, and repeats the cycle. The rectangular area covered by this scanning, is termed a **raster**.

Typically, there are 625 lines on the raster (or 1250, in a high definition system), and the cycle time is $\frac{1}{50}$ (or, in some countries, $\frac{1}{60}$) of a second. Instead of covering every line with every scan (frame), it is usual for a system of double or triple interlacing to be operated. This involves, in the case of double interlacing, coverage of alternate lines during one frame, followed by scanning of the intervening alternate lines. The complete picture is thus totally renewed every $\frac{1}{25}$ (or $\frac{1}{30}$) of a second – a rate which satisfies the retina of the eye's requirement for a continuous image.

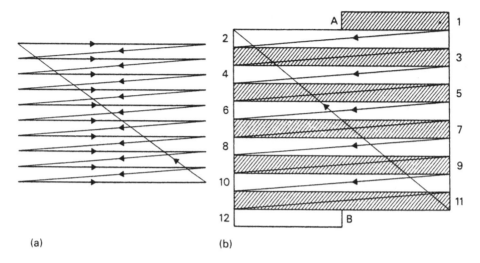

(a)                            (b)

**Fig. 7.13** Television scanning principle. In both the camera and the picture monitor tube, the focused, fine electron beam traces horizontal lines across the raster. After completing one frame, it flies back diagonally, to repeat the cycle. Instead of scanning every line (a), interlacing is performed so that either alternate lines (b) or every third line is scanned, in turn, during a lengthened cycle, until every line is covered.

When the electrons strike the photoconductive layer, they are conducted through to the signal electrode, from where they are collected by an outer, circular metallic ring. From here, they are conducted to an amplification system, to form the **video signal**. The significance of the photoconductive layer can now be appreciated. The rate at which the electrons pass through to the signal electrode depends on the brightness of the part of the mosaic through which they are passing. If it is brightly lit, corresponding to a light part of the image, conduction is easily achieved: the rate of flow – that is, the current – is high. If the mosaic part is dark, there will be opposition to conduction, restricting the current.

As the electron beam scans the image, therefore, a continuously varying current is produced – the video signal – conveying information about the image composition, line by line.

There are practical problems: stray, random electrons can interfere with the image, superimposing a flecked appearance on it, termed **noise**; and the phenomenon of **image persistence** – a residual ghosting, commonly known as **lag** – can inhibit the demonstration of rapid movements. Alternatives to the vidicon camera can present a different profile of problems. Another common camera type is the plumbicon, so-called because its photoconductor material is lead monoxide. This can cope better with rapid movement (it shows less lag). However, because it has less lag it shows more noise.

## 7.7 The television monitor

In the television monitor, an image is constructed to correspond to the original, relayed to it in the form of a video signal. Again, the monitor is based on an evacuated glass envelope, narrow and cylindrical at the back but flaring out to the familiar, wide viewing screen at the front. Again too, like the television camera, there is an electron source at the back of the tube. The electrons are accelerated forwards by a potential difference of about 20 kV. Controlling electrodes form the electrons into a fine, focused beam which impinges on a fluorescent layer lining the front of the envelope, according to a scanning cycle adjusted to synchronize exactly with the camera's.

The fluorescent screen, coated onto the inside of the front of the picture tube, is composed of phosphors, activators and *killers*, which ensure that the kinetic energy of the bombarding electrons is immediately and reliably converted into visible light. This is viewed from the exterior, as the reconstructed television image. As it traces out its path, the illuminated spot

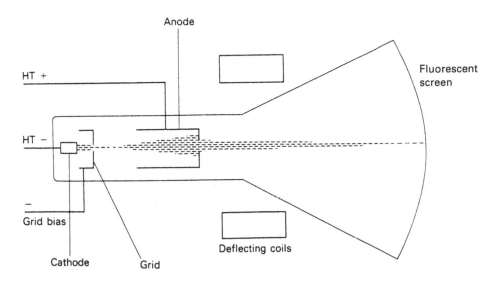

**Fig. 7.14** Principal features of a television picture monitor tube. The electron beam is controlled by deflection coils, to scan the fluorescent screen, recreating images from the video signal originated by the television camera.

which marks the position of the bombarding electron beam varies in brightness, according to electron intensity. A dense electron beam results in strong fluorescence; a sparse flow of electrons produces weak fluorescence.

The electron beam emitted from the filament passes through a control grid which has a focusing function but also a crucial role in the recreation of the televised image: it controls the rate at which electrons pass forward, to bombard the fluorescent screen. A highly negative potential severely restricts the rate at which electrons pass through, to create fluorescence on the screen; a less negative potential allows the flow to increase. The controlling influence, determining whether the electrons' passage is more or less intense, is derived from the video signal transmitted from the television camera. In this way, the video signal controls the varying brightness of fluorescence; the scanning beam thus copies the scanning pattern from the original image, onto the monitor's screen.

## 7.8 Image recording

There are two basic methods: photographic (now tending to become obsolete) and electronic (modern).

A fluorographic camera can record *single shot* still images of the fluoroscopic image or, for specialized use, a moving, cine image. The cameras are fed with the light beam from the image intensifier output, via the distributor.

The video signal is versatile. It can be recorded on magnetic tape or disc or fed to a *memory* device. This is extremely useful on occasions when the individuality of the projection, rather than the need for demonstrating movement, is required. An instance occurs frequently during surgery, when the surgeon wishes to study the fluoroscopic image but does not wish, at the same time, to be continuously exposing the patient (or nearby personnel) to an accumulating radiation hazard. A short segment of the video signal is recorded and continuously replayed to produce a static image on the monitor, until it is cancelled by progress to another, or to resume instantaneous imaging. Electronic image manipulation – enhancement and control – are possible when the video signal has been digitized. Although still in a development stage, digital imaging offers facilities which promise to revolutionize radiodiagnosis.

### *Automatic brightness/exposure control*

As the radiation field is moved around during fluoroscopy, to show different parts of the patient's body, the brightness of the screen image will tend to change: some parts of the body are more or less radiolucent than others. If these parts were to be radiographed separately, the radiographer would select different factors, to adjust the parameters of the X-ray beam – principally its quality. A similar change can be automatically prompted by a monitoring device which samples the brightness of the image emerging from the intensifier. This monitor can feed back either to the electrical supply to the X-ray tube (kV and/or mA) or to the television system's gain control.

If the kV and mA are varied, the radiation dose rate to the patient will also change, but the image quality and its diagnostic value will tend to remain constant. If the radiation quality and intensity are fixed, the dose rate to the patient will be constant (whether it is at a correct level or not), but the picture quality, through variability of gain, will tend to change.

## 7.9 Summary of intensified fluoroscopy

In view of its universal use, it seems unnecessary to consider the *advantages* of image intensification, compared with an obsolete alternative. Instead, it may be most helpful to summarize some aspects of its operation, by which a dynamic, X-ray image of the patient can be obtained.

The fluoroscopic facility – being able to see the object without the delays and uncertainties which attend radiography – can allow surgical and interventional examinations to be performed with reliability.

While fluoroscopy is in progress, the radiation dose rate to the patient is minimized by the efficiency of the energy conversion system – from X-rays to visible light.

Although some equipment is rather fixed in its adaptability to the patient, other units are very versatile, providing an imaging facility which is adjustable to every required situation.

Through its conversion to an electronic video signal, a range of options are available for displaying and processing the fluoroscopic image:

(1) It can be displayed simultaneously on several monitors, for multiple viewing, including transmission to a remote audience.
(2) It can be recorded and played back on standard video equipment.
(3) Most importantly, the video signal can be digitized and employed in a manipulative system, vastly extending the range of its clinical applications.

## 7.10 Follow-up practical

Being a modality which offers the opportunity to *watch* rather than just *see*, there is no substitute, in the student's progressive learning, for first-hand observation of fluoroscopic equipment, used in its various applications: from relatively simple gastro-intestinal examinations through to the complexities of cardiovascular and neurological interventions.

# Part Five
# Specialized Radiographic Equipment

The basic radiographic equipment described in Part Four is versatile: it can be used to carry out a wide range of examinations. For specialized procedures outside this range, however, specialized or *dedicated* equipment is required.

While it is possible in some instances for a ward patient, still in bed, to be taken to the hospital's imaging department, in others, such a journey may be out of the question. In such cases, and to provide X-ray imaging during procedures in the operating theatre, mobile equipment (Chapter 8) is needed.

The condition of a traumatized patient can lie anywhere within a range from slightly injured to totally disabled and unconscious. Patients with minor injuries may safely be radiographed with basic, general purpose equipment, but in more serious cases this is inadequate. The principle of arranging the equipment around the undisturbed patient can only be achieved with a specialized *accident system* (Chapter 9).

This same principle of matching equipment to the specialized needs of the radiographic examination governs the design of both dental (Chapter 10) and mammographic equipment (Chapter 11). In each case, there is not only a mechanical requirement for the equipment to fit a comfortably positioned patient, but also an electrical specialization, to produce X-rays of an appropriate quality.

To carry out conventional tomography, special mechanical linkage is required, with refined control over movement of X-ray tube and film. Equipment which can provide these facilities is described in Chapter 12.

# Chapter 8
# Mobile Radiographic Equipment

## 8.1 Introduction

Mobile X-ray equipment has a long history. It was conceived during the early days of radiography, as the obvious solution to providing facilities for:

(1) In-patients who could not leave their beds, especially those who could not be moved away from their wards.
(2) Surgeons who required *X-ray control* guidance during the course of their work in the operating theatre.

In common with X-ray equipment in general, technical innovations have improved the performance of mobile equipment, but its basic design has remained the same: a wheeled base onto which is built an X-ray generator with its control panel, and a supported X-ray tube.

It is ironic that, as its power has improved, mobile X-ray equipment may be required to perform fewer X-ray examinations than in previous years. Hospital in-patients are now rarely required to make an open air, outside journey from their wards to the imaging department; lifts (elevators) are routinely large enough to accommodate a hospital bed; and doorways and corridors are built with sensible width. Thus, many bedridden patients in need of radiography are now transferred safely from their wards to the imaging department, where they can be examined with all the efficiency that department can offer. These facilities include full radiation protection: for the patient, of course, but also for other personnel who otherwise, in the hospital ward, could have been at risk.

Strict radiation protection legislation is designed to provide safe control of radiographic procedures in a hospital ward. The exposure handswitch cable must be at least 2 m long, to allow the radiographer to stand distant from the irradiated patient, and mandatory precautions are laid down for protection of personnel not involved with the examination, but even these may not ensure that safety meets the standards provided in an imaging department.

The use of purely radiographic equipment in the operating theatre has declined since the introduction of mobile fluoroscopic equipment. The delay for all concerned, not least the anaesthetized patient, while radiographs were exposed, processed and returned to the theatre, has become a thing of the past due to the instant imaging which fluoroscopy can provide.

Despite these points, the services of mobile X-ray equipment can be in demand all day in a busy hospital. Study of the principal features of their construction and operation is necessary, as always, for correct and safe use.

## 8.2 Electrical energy sources

Permanently installed X-ray generators, receiving their energy from *mains* electrical supplies, are usually identified according to their output (tube) kilovoltage waveform, although this may also imply the nature of the mains input. In contrast, mobile equipment tends to be categorized by its energy input source – although, here again, there may be an implication: this time, of the tube waveform.

### *Tube voltage waveform*

Electrical energy, the *raw material* for conversion into X-rays, may be obtained in three different ways. Each has benefits to offer but each also has its shortcomings.

(1) Energy may be drawn for X-ray exposures directly from the mains voltage supply, as is the case with permanently installed, static generators. This is a convenience: there is no need for the energy to be carried around within the mobile equipment, but supply variations at different locations where the equipment is used can raise difficulties affecting image quality.

(2) A capacitor can be charged from the mains voltage to the required potential difference (kV) and then discharged through the X-ray tube. This can provide consistently reliable results, but the X-ray beam characteristics are unusual and there are limits to the level of output power which can be achieved.

(3) Battery design has improved up to a point at which both voltage and current supplies can satisfactorily provide the energy required by an X-ray generator. Such an arrangement enables equipment to be used freely, without the need for dependence on a mains supply. Regular recharging and careful maintenance are required, however, if operation is to be reliable.

## 8.3 Mains-dependent mobile equipment

### *Supply cable*

Mobile X-ray equipment which depends on a mains voltage supply must have a robust connection cable. This encloses three low resistance conductors, each with a relatively large cross-sectional area. Two of the conductors carry the current which the generator draws when an exposure is made. The third provides a safe, reliable connection to earth.

The cable must be long enough for the equipment to be used in most locations, provided there is a convenient mains outlet socket, but not so long that its resistance becomes significant. When not in use, the cable is wound onto a wheel-type storage drum built into the equipment, both for tidiness and protection against physical damage.

It should be noted that the use of extension cables is considered to be an unsafe practice. The extra length of cable and the interception of an extra plug and socket increase the resistance. This has two possible effects: it may significantly increase the voltage drop which occurs during an exposure and it may weaken the earth connection, reducing the safety of the equipment.

## 8.4 Conventional generators

### *Rating of the mains connection*

During an exposure, the current drawn from the mains by a mobile X-ray generator is commonly about 30 A and may be higher. This value is above the current drawn by most electrical appliances and probably higher than the maximum for which the electrical wiring and sockets in a hospital ward are rated. Normally, currents which exceed the rated maximum are cut off by the action of fuses or circuit breakers before the heat they produce can threaten the safety of the installation. X-ray exposures, however, are unusually brief, compared with the periods for which other electrical appliances operate. This fact leads to (and justifies) the commonest arrangement: the fuses employed are of a slow-acting type. The safety threat from the high current is quickly over and the X-ray examination can be satisfactorily concluded.

Normal plugs fitted to the supply cables or flexes of electrical equipment contain fuses. In the case of X-ray equipment, there is no point in having a plug fitted with a fuse: protection is provided by the fuses which guard the whole wiring circuit. The type of plug fitted to the mobile X-ray equipment cable, therefore, needs to be special. It must be robust, large enough to accommodate a thicker-than-average supply cable and easily identifiable. The red *Walsall* plug is an example.

### *Mains resistance compensation*

The high current drawn from the mains during an X-ray exposure inevitably causes a voltage drop to occur in the supply cable and also in the high tension transformer. Without compensation, this would pass on its effect to the tube kilovoltage and to the radiographic image (in its density and contrast). The voltage drop is proportional to both the current and the supply cable's resistance. Compensation circuitry is built into the generator, to counter the effect of the voltage drop. When an mA value is selected, the supply current is anticipated and an appropriate adjustment is made to the voltage tapped from the autotransformer, to maintain the tube kilovoltage at the required value.

The compensation will be accurate only with a particular value of mains resistance. The equipment manufacturers specify a value and design their compensation circuitry accordingly. It is then the responsibility of the installation engineers to ensure that this value actually applies. With a permanently installed generator, this task only needs to be carried out once. The on-site resistance is measured. If it exactly matches the specified value, no action is necessary. If on-site resistance is less than the specified value, the engineers make up the difference by inserting a series *padding* resistor. In the unlikely event of the on-site resistance being too high, rewiring of the supply is necessary.

In the case of mobile X-ray equipment, the radiographer is, in effect, the *installation engineer*. The first task to perform after plugging in the generator is to make a compensation, if required, for the mains resistance. There may be a control to operate in conjunction with a meter on the instrument panel; or an adjustment to make, to match a calibration value displayed on the mains (wall) socket.

If this compensation facility is provided, it is important that it is operated correctly, if radiographic image quality is to be reliable.

### Mains voltage compensation

This may be manual or automatic. If manual, the need for reliable image quality again demands careful and accurate adjustment.

### Rectification

Operating (exposing) from a mains socket, only single-phase generators are encountered. These may be of the conventional two-pulse type or, increasingly, of the middle frequency *multi-pulse* type.

A two-pulse generator has its high tension components (transformers and rectifiers) housed in a compact tank on the wheeled base, supplying a standard, rotating anode X-ray tube via high tension cables.

A middle frequency generator may have all its high tension components together with the X-ray tube, inside an enlarged housing, fed from the control panel by a single, low tension flex.

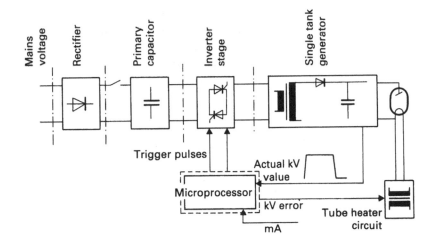

**Fig. 8.1** Principle of operation of a high frequency generator. A microprocessor monitors and ensures accuracy of kilovoltage and tube current. The combination of transformers and tube insert within a single tank is a particularly important feature of a mobile unit. (*By courtesy of Siemens plc.*)

The two-pulse generator will require mains compensation circuitry for accurate operation. The middle frequency generator is likely to incorporate electronic feedback devices and microprocessors, which monitor tube output and make it independent of mains variations.

## 8.5 Capacitor discharge equipment

The principle advantage of producing X-rays from the energy stored in and then discharged from a capacitor is consistency. With given exposure factors, results are reproduced identically, time after time. Mains voltage and resistance variations only have their effects upon the act of charging the capacitor, which takes place just before the X-ray exposure is made. Such effects are irrelevant.

When an exposure is required, the method of operation, in outline, is that the radiographer selects values of kV and mAs. The switch is then operated to charge the capacitor to the required kilovoltage, via the high tension generator. The X-ray exposure involves first disconnecting the capacitor from its high tension supply and then connecting it across the X-ray tube. A special type of X-ray tube is required, which incorporates a third electrode – a *grid* interposed between cathode and anode – which is at a high negative potential or *bias*. The effect of the negative bias is to prevent filament electrons from crossing to the anode. Connection of the capacitor to the tube therefore has no immediate effect. The exposure begins when the negative bias is removed and is ended when the bias is reimposed.

At the end of the timed exposure, when the required charge (mAs) has crossed the tube, the negative grid bias is reimposed to prevent further conduction. The capacitor is then disconnected from the tube and discharged, with no effect.

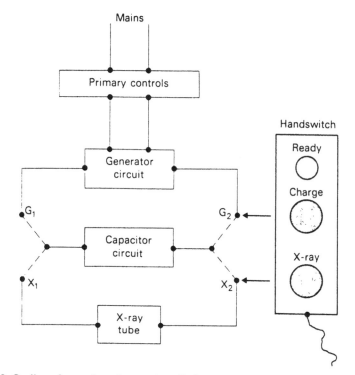

**Fig. 8.2** Outline of operation of a capacitor-discharge generator. Prior to exposure, switches $X_1$ and $X_2$ are open. $G_1$ and $G_2$ are closed by the charge control. Operation of the X-ray exposure control opens $G_1$ and $G_2$ to isolate the charged capacitor, then closes $X_1$ and $_x2$, to discharge it through the X-ray tube.

It is relevant to remember that the milliampere second is a unit of electric charge, known outside radiography as a millicoulomb (mC). The capacitance of a capacitor – its ability to store electric charge – is not measured in absolute terms (i.e. in millicoulombs), but as the ratio between the charge stored on its plates and the potential difference between them. The unit of capacitance, the farad, indicates a storage of 1 coulomb per volt: in practical terms, a very large capacitance.

The capacitor employed in mobile X-ray equipment usually has a capacitance of 1 microfarad, which means that every mC of charge stored on its plates creates a potential difference of 1 kV across it. When discharged, therefore, the potential difference falls by 1 kV for every mC – i.e. every mAs – of the exposure. For example, a selected exposure of 90 kV and 20 mAs results in a final potential difference across the tube of 70 kV. This fact highlights the deficiency of capacitor discharge as a means of producing X-rays: during the exposure, the beam's quality and intensity both fall. Selection of exposure factors, particularly the starting kilovoltage, must therefore be made very carefully, in order to produce the required object penetration, object and density.

In producing a beam of varying quality and intensity, the discharging capacitor may be said to produce similar results to a pulsating kilovoltage – i.e. one which varies between its peak and zero. In that the capacitor's potential difference is not allowed to fall to values even close to zero, its performance may actually be considered better than a pulsing supply. This fall in kilovoltage imposes a limit on the usable mAs, however. If a large mAs is selected, therefore, it must be remembered that the kV will undergo a proportionate drop, and the eventual quality of the X-ray beam may be too low for image formation. In this case, it would contribute only to the dose to the patient.

Capacitor discharge operation raises an interesting and important question regarding tube filament temperature. Receiving its energy from a capacitor, the tube does not operate according to normal practice, where filament temperature dictates the value of tube current. The tube current will decay exponentially, as the capacitor discharges. The effect of filament temperature will be, through making electrons more or less plentiful, to give the tube a particular value of electrical resistance. This property will control the rate of flow of charge, i.e. the rate of X-ray production. Significantly, it also therefore controls the rate of production of heat. In order to protect the anode against a risk of thermal damage, the tube filament temperature may be automatically controlled, according to the amount of heat which will be produced during the exposure: for larger exposures, the temperature may be reduced, to slow down the rate of discharge.

## 8.6 Battery-powered generators

The use of batteries as the energy source is a convenience which has few disadvantages, provided that correct, regular charging procedures are observed, to keep the batteries in full working order. Their direct voltage output has first to be converted into an alternating voltage, so that it can be transformed into a kilovoltage. This is then followed by rectification: conversion of the alternating kilovoltage into a unidirectional waveform for application across the X-ray tube. At first sight these steps may seem contradictory, but it must be remembered that without conversion to an alternating form, stepping up of the voltage could not be achieved.

Depending on the equipment, the kilovoltage applied across the tube may be virtually a direct voltage; at the stage of converting the battery output into an alternating voltage, there is no obligation to conform to mains voltage frequency: much higher frequencies can be produced, to enhance efficiency.

The batteries may be nickel-cadmium or the more conventional lead-acid type. All batteries are sealed for safety. Charging is achieved by connecting the generator to a mains voltage supply at times when it is not required for radiography. During these periods, security is essential: no unauthorized person must be allowed access to the equipment, either to interfere with the charging process or to undergo risk of personal harm.

## 8.7 X-ray tubes

The power available from modern mobile generators is wasted if the X-ray tube is not fitted with a rotating anode. In some situations, the anode may usefully be *high speed*, to take advantage of the generator's facilities.

Capacitor discharge equipment units have X-ray tubes which incorporate a grid, to switch exposures, and are linked to their high tension supply via special, four-conductor cables.

Some tubes may be incorporated with their high tension circuitry in a *single tank* type of housing. This is bulkier than a simple tube but, requiring only a low voltage feed, offers the advantage of freedom from cumbersome, high tension cables.

X-ray tubes are invariably fitted with LBD units. Scales and angle indicators are fitted to guide radiographers towards accuracy, as they perform examinations in non-standard and sometimes adverse conditions.

The X-ray tube is the most delicate (and expensive) component of a mobile equipment unit. It is essential that it is protected against physical damage, particularly when the unit is in motion, by being locked into a protected recess or in some other firmly supported position.

## 8.8 Physical features

### The wheeled base

Unfortunately for those who have to move the mobile unit and manoeuvre it around within a restricted space, there is a requirement for the base on which the unit is built to be weighty. This gives the equipment its essential stability, particularly when it has to counteract the levering action of a fully extended tube support.

The wheels are fitted with tyres made from antistatic rubber, for safety.

## The drive unit

The trend in X-ray generator design towards space reduction has been followed in mobile equipment design, no less than in large, permanent units. The space saved by a smaller generator has not led directly to a reduction in the size of a mobile unit, however. More often than not, it has been taken as an opportunity for fitting a motorized drive unit. This is at least a convenience and may be considered to be essential, both in time saving and in eliminating the risk of strain injuries to staff who have to move the equipment from place to place.

The motor should offer forward and reverse controls, at both slow and faster speeds. Its batteries (which may either also provide energy for exposures or be separate) need to be charged regularly and in protected circumstances, for safety.

Matching the motor drive in their efficiency must be appropriate brakes and locks, by which the equipment can be slowed and immobilized.

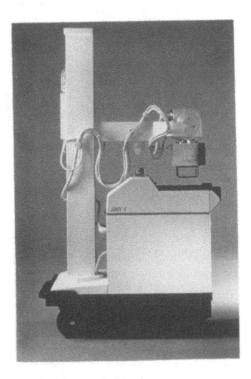

**Fig. 8.3** A mobile radiographic unit with the tube on a cross-arm, mounted on a vertical column. (*By courtesy of IGE Medical Systems.*)

## Tube support

A fundamental requirement is for the tube to be supported safely and to offer the radiographer a range of adjustable movements and positions which enable techniques to be performed easily, particularly if working space is restricted. There may be a vertical column with a cross-arm on which the tube is mounted. Alternatively, there may be a stout, multi-jointed arm arising from the base which is held in its adjusted position by friction.

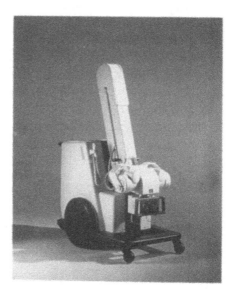

Fig. 8.4 A mobile radiographic unit with the tube mounted on a multi-jointed extension arm. (*By courtesy of IGE Medical Systems.*)

## Security

By being free for movement around the hospital, mobile X-ray equipment is at greater risk of damage, abuse and contamination than the permanent equipment in locked rooms in the imaging department.

Mobile equipment must be lockable, that is it should be capable of being rendered stationary and unusable, except by an authorized member of staff who possesses the appropriate key.

When *parked*, mobile equipment should be safe from access by patients and visitors, ideally in a locked or secluded place. Regular cleaning is required and this task can be simplified by the use of protective dustproof covers.

## 8.9 Follow-up practical

Student radiographers, on the whole, are soon introduced to the pleasures of handling mobile X-ray equipment. The process of evaluation – comparing one unit's strengths and weaknesses with another's – therefore probably begins quite early during their training. This should be on an increasing scientific basis, as the course progresses, bringing in some of the points raised during this chapter.

# Chapter 9
# Accident and Emergency X-Ray Equipment

## 9.1 Introduction

The majority of examinations carried out in accident and emergency (A & E) imaging departments involve cases of simple trauma. An A & E department may also be used for general radiography, however, taking the workload of a main imaging department, outside normal working hours. X-ray equipment for A & E must therefore be able to deal satisfactorily with general requests, as well as with more complex, severe trauma cases.

Professional opinion tends to be divided on the matter of ideal equipment for A & E procedures. There are those who believe that high quality radiographs are achievable while the patient remains on an accident trolley, but others who believe that all patients must be moved onto a standard examination couch which incorporates a moving grid.

The central features of any system designed to examine seriously injured patients are:

(1) That the patient should be required to move as little as possible during the examination.
(2) Radiography in any plane should be possible.
(3) The examination should be performed in the shortest possible time.
(4) The dose to the patient must be as low as is reasonably achievable.

Isocentric units for skeletal radiography, with specialized, variable height tables, are now generally recognized as the *state of the art* choice for trauma radiography. The commonest alternative is a system such as the *Patient Care System* (Picker), which does not require movement of the patient from the trolley at all. The other widely used method, that of moving the patient from a trolley onto an X-ray table, is improved by a patient transfer system such as a sliding mattress.

Additionally, there are other items of equipment and accessories of particular value to radiographers in A & E X-ray rooms.

## 9.2 Basic trolley design

Whatever system is in use, the trolley must have certain common characteristics to make it suitable for transporting severely injured patients:

(1)  A means to tilt the trolley top.

(2)  A variable height adjustment, to allow resuscitation and access.

(3)  An adjustable backrest which can be inclined at various angles.

(4)  Side rests (cot sides) which can be raised and lowered as necessary.

(5)  A drip stand holder.

(6)  An oxygen bottle holder.

(7)  Brakes on the wheels and steering locks.

(8)  A radiolucent, rubber covered foam mattress, capable of being detached to slide across onto an X-ray table.

(9)  Easily cleaned, chemical resistant surfaces.

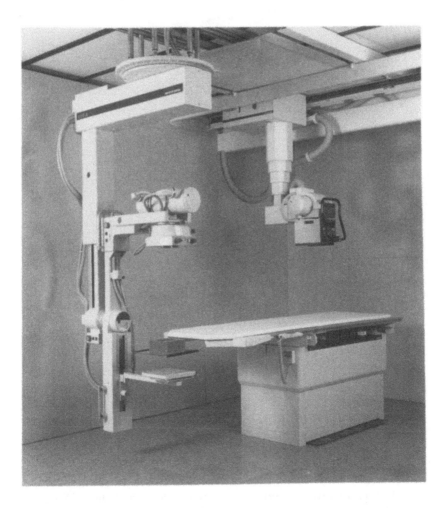

**Fig. 9.1** Isocentric equipment for skeletal radiography. The ceiling-mounted unit can be moved around the patient, supported on a radiolucent table, to produce standardized radiographic projections without need to move the patient. (*Courtesy of Siemens plc.*)

## 9.3 Isocentric skull unit with variable height table

The equipment comprises:

(1) A trolley with a sliding mattress capable of being moved onto the associated X-ray table.
(2) A ceiling-mounted tube with a linked film holder for skull and facial radiography.

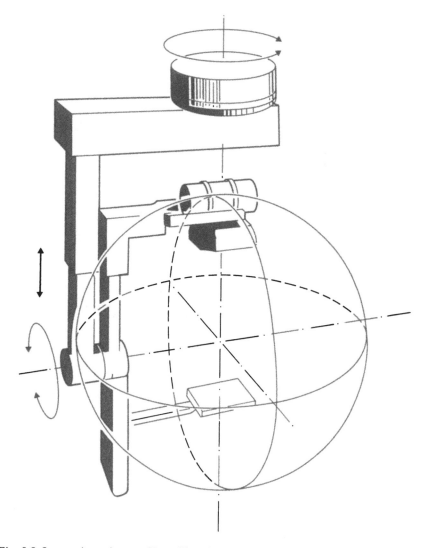

**Fig. 9.2** Isocentric equipment. Versatility of multi-plane rotation of X-ray tube and linked film support is offered. Techniques involve positioning this equipment in relation to the patient, so that the rotation isocentre coincides with the structure being examined. Multi-plane angulations/projections can then be achieved without need to move the patient from an original, rest position. (*By courtesy of Siemens plc.*)

(3) A variable height table with extending head rest and linked table top drive.

(4) A microprocessor controlled generator with anatomical programming.

(5) A ceiling mounted tube fitment for skeletal radiography.

The basic design of the trolley has been previously described. The isocentric skull unit incorporates an X-ray tube centred and linked to a film holder fitted with a stationary grid. The unit is designed to allow an infinite range of angles to be selected. It is mounted so that it is free to rotate around a common fulcrum. A central point within the patient's skull is adjusted to coincide with this fulcrum. Once in this *reference position*, usually supine, no further movement of the patient is necessary: the tube and film holder are rotated around until the X-ray beam is angled as required for any given projection.

The variable height table is designed to allow ease of access, being adjustable to the height of the trolley. It can also be lowered to allow easy access for patients who are unable to climb from a step onto the table. The table top is linked by motorized movements to the cranial unit so that fine adjustments of the patient's position can be made, especially for the more sophisticated isocentric skull techniques which can also be carried out on this unit. Skull radiography is made particularly convenient by the provision of a radiolucent, narrow extending head rest.

The ceiling-mounted tube fitment allows for radiography of the rest of the trunk and upper and lower limbs. With the patient moved down on the mattress slightly, horizontal beam techniques, so often essential in trauma radiography, can be performed with ease.

The X-ray generator which supplies this unit should have a high frequency, high power output, with anatomical programming and automatic exposure control.

## 9.4 Trolley-based system

The most commonly encountered system is the *Care System*, which allows simple skull radiography and complete skeletal radiography without moving the patient from the trolley. This system is particularly useful where radiographers are working single-handed or cannot easily obtain assistance to move patients safely onto an X-ray table. This system also tends to increase efficiency, as examinations can generally be carried out in a significantly shorter time.

The trolley has a long slot suitable for the insertion of either a film with an attached grid or the purpose-built gridded film carrier. By allowing positioning of the film in any required orientation, examinations such as of the

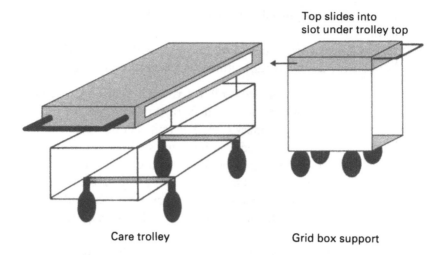

Top slides into
slot under trolley top

Care trolley                    Grid box support

**Fig. 9.3** Principle of the *Care* trolley system.

abdomen, pelvis or vertebral column can be performed with relative ease.

Apart from the trolley, the other essential components of the system are:

(1) a mobile cassette carrier; and
(2) an optical light beam positioning unit, fitted in relation to a ceiling-suspended X-ray tube.

The mobile cassette carrier is a cabinet which provides easy transport of the gridded cassette unit and storage of films or accessories, as necessary. The cassette unit can thus be inserted simply into the trolley by drawing the holder up to the side of the unit, operating the control lever and applying slight pressure in a forward direction. The trolley thus becomes converted easily and effectively into a simple X-ray table.

The optical link is provided by two lights fixed to the X-ray tube's mounting or the LBD. These are orientated so that when they converge on a cut-out square on the cassette unit, the film is centred and the focus–film distance is correct.

Although in theory a moving grid is considered essential if radiographs are to be unaffected by grid lines, the images produced by these trolley-based units can be of an equally high quality, provided that the correct techniques are employed. (A similar standard can be obtained from the isocentric system for skull radiography which also has a fixed grid system and is, as previously mentioned, widely considered to be *state of the art*.

## 9.5 Trauma resuscitation room

The most commonly used X-ray equipment in a resuscitation room is a mobile X-ray set. Critical features of this equipment when used in the resuscitation room are high power, ease of movement and reliable output. A capacitor-discharge unit is ideal, providing consistent exposures, despite simultaneous use of a range of other electrical equipment within the same area.

### Dedicated equipment

In many large trauma units a dedicated X-ray examination facility is located within the resuscitation room. There are various configurations.

A ceiling-mounted tube may be installed, with a generator and control panel, for operation in exactly the same way as a unit located in a conventional X-ray room. Thus, for the purposes of radiation protection, the resuscitation room is a designated area. The advantage of such units is that they allow for the speedy production of the three radiographs now widely recognized as being essential for the management of multiple trauma (an anteroposterior pelvis, a chest radiograph and a lateral cervical spine) whilst other resuscitation measures are being undertaken. Otherwise, the crowd of medical and nursing staff found, of necessity, in the resuscitation area, make access difficult for a wheeled mobile X-ray set.

If a light linked cassette carrier and a *Care* type trolley, as previously described, are available, these can be used successfully in the resuscitation area. The light centring fitment is fixed to either the mobile X-ray set or the dedicated ceiling mounted tube.

## 9.6 Ancillary equipment

In the dedicated casualty X-ray room, some other items of equipment will be regularly used and a brief mention is therefore included.

### Orthopantomograph

This makes an excellent addition to the equipment of an accident and emergency room. It can be used quickly and easily to provide detailed information concerning injuries to the mandible. This may frequently be needed in most accident centres to complement other views of the face. It should be noted, however, that the patient must be able to co-operate for an orthopantomograph examination to be carried out.

### Lateral cassette holder

This piece of equipment will find frequent use. One simple design consists of a wheeled unit with an angular arm which can be moved into various angles and adjusted to support most sizes of cassette. The cassette holder is located at the end of the extending arm, thus the film can be tilted to suit the required projection. This equipment can be used for horizontal beam projections quite successfully.

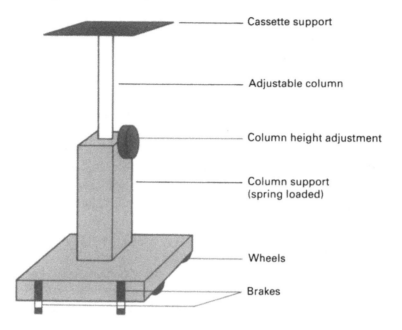

Fig. 9.4 Mobile horizontal cassette support.

### Horizontal cassette support

A mobile cassette support with a sheet metal top, a rubber surface and variable height adjustment is an invaluable aid for radiography of a patient confined to a trolley. It allows cassettes to be laid next to a patient for radiography of the hand or forearm, or supported for horizontal beam projections.

### Stationary grids

A range of stationary grids are regularly required for horizontal beam lateral views – of the spine, for example.

### Patient transfer aids

Of the aids in general use, one type is made of a cylinder of material which will roll with a patient, while being gently edged across from trolley to table. The other design consists of a fibreglass board with a slippery surface. This allows patients to be slid from trolley to mattress and back again as necessary.

## 9.7 Follow-up practical

Pay visits to A & E imaging departments in separate hospitals, which are equipped with different radiography systems, to study the relative advantages which each system offers and its implications for radiographic techniques.

# Chapter 10
# Equipment for Dental Radiography

## 10.1 Intra-oral equipment

Dental equipment for intra-oral X-ray examinations (when the film is placed inside the patient's mouth) is, from one perspective, basic rather than specialized. It is comparable with equipment at an early stage of development for general radiography. Its low power – a moderately low kilovoltage and a low tube current – is still sufficient to meet the demands of dental radiography. Only modest penetration is required and with the short focus–film distance, a relatively weak tube output intensity is acceptable.

Low power of X-ray production implies a relatively low rate of heat production – sufficiently so to lie within the safe capability of a stationary anode X-ray tube, operating in self-rectification conditions. These specifications can be met by *single tank* construction: X-ray tube and high tension circuitry combined within a single, shockproofed housing.

This design easily matches the ideal physical requirements for intra-oral dental radiography: a light and compact tube, easily manoeuvred around the patient's face.

The dental tube head contains a stationary anode tube insert, high tension transformer and tube filament transformer. It is mounted on a device, termed a gimbal, which allows rotation in two planes. Scales are incorporated to indicate angles of rotation, as required for dental radiographic techniques.

The tube port is fitted with a cone which collimates and centres the X-ray beam, and guides the radiographer to use the correct focus–film distance. The tube's inherent filtration is supplemented by added filtration at the tube port, to bring the total up to 1–2 mm of aluminium.

The tube head is insulated internally with oil, similar to a general-purpose X-ray tube, and its housing is lead lined and earthed via both its supply cable and its mounting. The tube is supported by a multi-jointed arm. The joints are loose enough to be flexed by slight pressure, but tight enough to hold by friction, at the set angulations.

The arm also supports or may enclose the cable which supplies the high tension and filament transformer primary windings. This is only a low voltage (*low tension*) supply, not requiring the bulky, restricting high tension

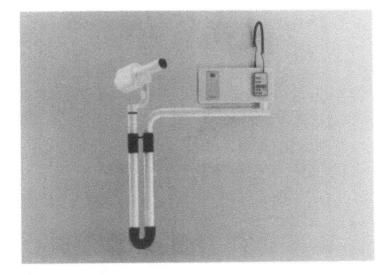

**Fig. 10.1** Dental X-ray unit. A modern unit for intra-oral dental radiography. The stationary anode X-ray tube has a 0.7 mm focal spot and is mounted at the rear of the single-tank head assembly. This arrangement lengthens the focus-object distance, to help minimize geometric unsharpness. The generator supplies a multipulse 60 kV or 70 kV waveform, a tube current of 7 mA and exposure times ranging from 0.01 s to 3.2 s. All compensation functions are automatic. Anatomical programming selection is shown on the handset. (*By courtesy of Siemens plc.*)

cables which normally supply an X-ray tube. This feature is significant in allowing the tube to be manoeuvrable. The support arm arises from a firm base which can be wall-mounted, ceiling-suspended or on a mobile, wheeled pedestal. These options account for regular or occasional use, in an X-ray room or dental surgery.

The tube supply cable emerges from and the mains voltage is fed to, a control panel or box. The principal control is an exposure timer. Some choice of kilovoltage may be offered but since, from patient to patient, the object density is fairly constant, the value is commonly fixed, at about 65 kV. Tube current also is usually fixed. If focal spot size is 0.6–0.8 mm, 10 mA is a typical value. X-ray output is thus varied by selection of shorter or longer exposure times.

The fixing of kV and mA values makes conventional display indicators unnecessary. A neon light on the control panel and/or on the tube head, and an audible buzz, may be the indicators that the tube is energized, during exposures. The exposure handswitch is on a flexible lead which permits the operator to stand at a maximum distance from the tube while it is energised, behind a protective screen and facing the patient, to ensure that the request for immobilization is being followed.

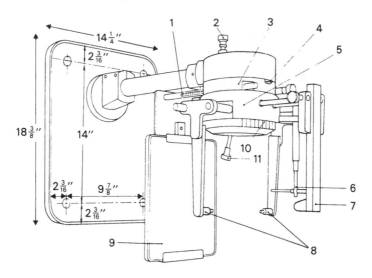

**Fig. 10.2** A craniostat. (*By courtesy of IGE Medical Systems.*)

1 Scale to indicate the distance between the median plane – or the midcoronal plane – of the head and cassette.
2 Lock for rotating head.
3 Cassette support which can be rotated through 360°.
4 Lock for cassette support.
5 Head rotates through 360° with four stop positions.

6 Orbital indicator.
7 Nasal positioner.
8 Ear locators.
9 Cassette.
10 Scale indicating the distance between the ear locators.
11 Control for adjusting the ear locators.

## 10.2 Cephalostat (craniostat)

This equipment is used in orthodontic practice. It enables standardized, accurate projections, most typically the *true lateral*, to be taken of the patient's head. The equipment permits both skull and facial soft tissue to be demonstrated, magnification to be calculated, and examinations to be reproduced and repeated exactly in the case of patients who are re-examined during the course of orthodontic treatment.

The cephalostat's accuracy and reliability is founded on its rigid wall mounting. This standardizes its position in relation to the X-ray tube, and the internal cassette and patient locations in relation to each other. The patient is located by ear plugs and a nasal positioner. A radiopaque scale aligned along the patient's median plane casts a magnified calibration on lateral radiographs.

A wedge, compensation filter of low density metal, duralmin, can be positioned to overlie facial soft tissue. This enables the radiograph simultaneously to show facial contours, cartilaginous and bony structures. A fine-line grid may be used focused to the tube distance, typically 140 cm. The X-ray tube is ideally a medium power rotating anode type, permanently fixed in relation to the cephalostat. The extended focus–film distance reduces geometric unsharpness and, although correction factors can be calculated, also lessens image magnification and the potentially misleading impressions which it can otherwise give.

## 10.3 Orthopantomography

As pointed out in the previous editions of this book, this term (commonly abbreviated to OPG or OPT) derives from the trade name for equipment manufactured by Siemens plc. Its adoption here is a recognition of widespread usage among radiographers and dentists. When analysed, this term indicates a correctness in the image's representation of its object – particularly interdental relationships; a panoramic rather than localized field; and demonstration of a slice of the patient's head rather than its whole.

Students are advised not to look for tomographic principles, however: this is a scanning technique, cleverly adapted to the complicated anatomical plan of the dental arches and their relations.

The X-ray tube and cassette are linked so that they move simultaneously, but in opposed directions, about a central pivot. The object does not coincide with this pivot, however (as it would in true tomography); it lies close to the film, following the principles of conventional radiographic imaging. During the exposure, the cassette moves around the face, from one ear to the other, while the X-ray tube swings around the head, posteriorly.

To achieve close and comfortable contact with the face, the cassette and the film within it are curved. As the exposure proceeds, the cassette is rotated around its centre of curvature. Contrary to what might be suspected, the film's curvature prevents image distortion, rather than being its cause; and film rotation has no motional effect on the image. The reason for both these points lies in the fact that the film is exposed through a narrow slit in a protective metal sheet. The image is built up from a sequence of parallel, exposed strips which are spread across the film from one end to the other, together making up a composite of the whole of the dental arches.

Scanning is most accurately performed when the X-ray beam moves along or across the object plane, maintaining a right-angled relationship throughout its travel. The curves of the dental arches – slight in the region of the temporomandibular joints, molar and premolar teeth; more marked anteriorly in the canine-incisor-canine region – account for the pivoting pattern of tube/film movement.

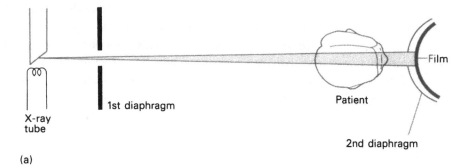

(a)

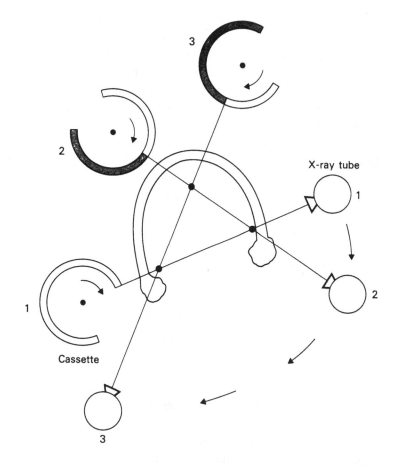

(b)

**Fig. 10.3** Panoramic dental equipment. (a) The X-ray beam is collimated at the tube head. Aligned to the centre of the beam is an aperture through which the film is exposed in its curved cassette, as the cassette rotates. (b) Plan view to show the synchronized pivoting movements of the X-ray tube and film: successive pivots ensure that the X-ray beam remains at right-angles to the varying curves of the dental arches.

During the exposure, tube and film rotate, in turn, about three points. The first gives a wide radius scan along one lateral part of the dental arch. The radius is then shortened by a second pivot, closer to the increased, anterior curvature. Finally, the pivot reverts to a lateral point, symmetrical with the first, to complete the scan. It is essential that the X-ray beam is very tightly collimated into a narrow *fan* shape by a slit aperture at the tube head. This minimizes the radiation hazard to the patient. Alignment to the slit aperture through which the beam exposes the film is essential for allowing the fan thickness to be minimized, and critical to the continuity of image formation. The slit through which the beam emerging from the patient passes, to expose the film, has a similarity (although on a larger scale) to one of the radiolucent channels within a grid. It allows free transmission of the primary beam but, by its depth – in this case, the thickness of the protective metal sheet – absorbs some of the oblique, non-aligned scattered radiation. It thus helps to maintain image contrast.

The exposure, with its tube and film movements, takes several seconds to complete. Naturally, therefore, comfort and immobilization of the patient are essential. The patient may either sit or stand, usually according to preference, and the vertical height of the whole assembly is adjustable, to match the patient. Nervous patients who are particularly daunted by the prospect of moving machinery may have its safety demonstrated to them beforehand – without an exposure – by the radiographer.

Positioning within the unit is made accurate, as in the cephalostat, by reference points and immobilization aids. These include a chin support, bite block, forehead support and additional lateral support. In addition, handles are available for the patient to grasp, to steady the body.

The length of an OPT exposure – maybe up to 15 seconds – has another implication: for the type of X-ray tube. Kilovoltages may typically be in the range 50–90 kV, but the tube current is low: 10–15 mA. There is thus a relatively low rate of X-ray and heat production, spread over a long time, and there are intervals between exposures imposed by the particular care needed for positioning and adjusting each patient. This requires a tube performance within the capability of a stationary anode. Physically, the compact form of a stationary anode tube allows freer access to the unit; and its lower weight than a rotating anode tube imposes a lower stress on the unit's drive mechanism. The focal spot size is typically 0.6 mm and total filtration 3 mm aluminium.

The slit diaphragm which collimates the beam can be adjusted in width for adults and children. A relatively short focus–film distance and necessary separation between the patient's face and the cassette lead to an image unsharpness of the teeth which is greater than with intra-oral techniques. There is also a magnification but the factor, typically 1.4, can be calculated if necessary for prosthetic procedures.

## 10.4 Follow-up practical

(1) Study carefully the pivoting movement of the orthopantomograph tube and film during a test run with no exposure. Its smoothness will tend to conceal the transfer from pivot to pivot.

(2) Compare this procedure with other scanning techniques you may have seen. Look for similarities between the two.

# Chapter 11
# Mammographic Equipment

## 11.1 Introduction

Mammographic techniques present two technical challenges which conventional, general purpose, X-ray equipment is unable to meet. First, the anatomical site and shape of the breasts makes their isolation more difficult than most other parts of the body. Second, the breast is composed of tissues which are markedly more radiolucent than most other structures within the body and which, in their composition, contrast with each other to a very limited extent.

Surrounding the practice of mammography are three important principles. These are not unique – they are relevant to other radiographic techniques – but they may be regarded as having heightened significance:

(1) The need to minimize the radiation hazard to the patient, especially in view of the breast's radiosensitivity.
(2) The requirement for image quality to be of a very high standard: detection of malignant changes may depend on identification of microcalcifications within the breast tissue.
(3) Emotional and physical care of the patient. Due to well organized health education, most patients attending for mammography are fully aware of the common purpose of the examination – the search for signs of malignant change – and are fully aware of the potential consequences of an unfavourable diagnosis. Patients may also anticipate, more so than during most other radiographic examinations, a degree of discomfort.

While the ability to cope with these considerations is one of the radiographer's skills, it should be recognized that there is a part which can be played by the equipment.

There are the technical requirements for radiation protection and image quality to be produced. If, as well as these, however, the equipment's appearance and mode of operation is non-threatening – if, for instance, its surfaces which come into contact with the patient are gently curved and warm to the touch, and its movements smooth and silent – the equipment can assist the radiographer in her work.

*Coverage of the whole breast*

For diagnostic reliability, mammographic images must demonstrate the whole of the breast, posteriorly as far as the thoracic wall. Mammographic units therefore incorporate a support plate or table for the breast, permanently linked and centred to an X-ray tube. This tube/plate assembly must be fully adjustable, to accommodate in comfort, patients of all heights. It must also be capable of being rotated for both vertical and horizontal beam projections.

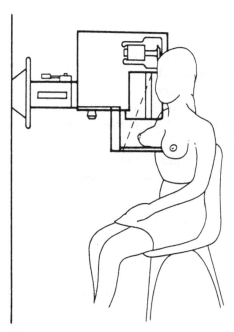

**Fig. 11.1** Mammographic unit showing breast supported on plate linked and centred to X-ray tube. (*By courtesy of Siemens plc.*)

*Demonstration of breast tissue*

The relative radiolucency of breast tissue demands an X-ray beam of low quality or penetrating power, compared with a beam used for other radiographic purposes. This implies the use of an unusually low X-ray tube kilovoltage. The generator which supplies energy to the tube must therefore offer a range of kV values extending lower than in the case of a general purpose generator – typically between 20 and 45 kV.

Unfortunately, the use of low kilovoltages has another effect on the X-ray beam, other than reducing its quality. X-ray beam intensity is directly proportional to the squared value of the tube kilovoltage. Thus at low kilovoltages there is a relatively low beam intensity. This fact has implications for the length of exposure times and raises the risk of increased movement unsharpness.

To offset this problem, wherever possible, a constant potential generator is employed; the focus–film distance is typically between 45 and 60 cm (less than for general radiographic techniques). This necessitates the use of a very fine focal spot, to maintain minimal geometric unsharpness (0.4 – 0.6 mm is typical), but this itself lowers the tube's rating, compared with larger focal spot sizes. There are, therefore, other constructional and design features of the mammographic X-ray tube which enhance the production of X-rays, to maintain beam intensity.

## 11.2 Mammographic X-ray tubes

### *Target and filter materials*

An important special feature of mammographic tubes is the optional use of molybdenum as the target material, in preference to tungsten. Considering molybdenum's lower atomic number, 42, compared with tungsten's 74, this appears to be a backward step, because the intensity of bremsstrahlung will be proportionately lower. This is offset by an advantage concerned with molybdenum's characteristic X-ray emission.

Whereas a potential difference across the tube of at least 70 kV is needed to produce *k* characteristic X-rays from a tungsten target, molybdenum's characteristic radiation can be produced by tube kilovoltages within the range used for mammography. Its presence in the X-ray beam greatly increases the intensity at the photon energy values needed for mammography. A recently introduced alternative target material is rhodium, which has an atomic number of 45. Its characteristic radiation has photon energies slightly higher than molybdenum's – favouring its use for imaging slightly denser breast tissue.

**Table 11.1** Comparison between characteristic photon energies emitted from tungsten and molybdenum targets.

| Target material | Electron binding energies (keV) | | Average characteristic photon energies for L to K transitions (keV) |
|---|---|---|---|
| | K Shell | L Shell | |
| Tungsten | 69.5 | 11.5 (average) | 58.0 |
| Molybdenum | 20.0 | 2.7 (average) | 17.0 |

Radiation protection legislation requires diagnostic X-ray beams to be filtered. The intention is to remove low energy photons from the beam which are incapable of reaching the image plane. Such radiation only increases the hazards to which the patient is potentially exposed.

Filtration of the low quality X-ray beam used for mammography presents particular difficulties. If practised routinely, it would seem to be a counterproductive factor, reducing the beam's intensity further below what is already a low level. This problem may be addressed by the use of materials other than aluminium (the routine for diagnostic filters), being very neatly solved by the use of the target metal again – this time as the filter material.

Photoelectric absorption of X-ray energy is inversely proportional to approximately the cubed value of photon energy. Absorption does not follow a smooth reduction, however, as photon energy increases: it is marked by recurrent temporary increases – so-called **absorption edges**. These occur when the rising value of photon energy reaches the shell binding energy values of the absorbing material. These edges indicate shell-by-shell increases in the number of tightly-bound electrons with which incident photons can interact. Just before they occur, however, at photon energy values just less than the shells' binding energies, photoelectric absorption has fallen to a low level. In other words, at these photon energy values, X-ray transmission is relatively efficient.

The characteristic radiation emitted from an element used as an X-ray tube target material naturally has a value slightly less than its own shell

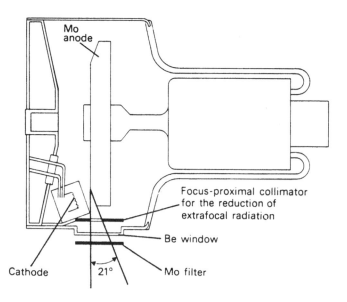

**Fig. 11.2** Longitudinal section through mammographic X-ray tube. (*By courtesy of Siemens plc.*)

binding energies. It thus follows that characteristic X-ray photons experience relatively little absorption when passing through a filter made of the same element that was used for the tube target.

The use of a molybdenum filter, for example, coupled with a molybdenum X-ray tube target, thus achieves the general purpose of removing from the beam the low energy, non-image-forming bremsstrahlung photons, but allows transmission of the significant, image-forming, characteristic X-radiation. Its action may be supported by minimization of the less selective inherent filtration – by thinning the glass envelope at the exit point of the *useful beam* or by fitting the tube with a window of beryllium (atomic number 4), which is less absorbent than glass. The benefits of molybdenum as a filter material are particularly apparent at kilovoltages between 20 and 25 kV. At higher values, as mentioned, tubes may have filters fitted which are made of rhodium or palladium.

### Electrode spacing

At low kilovoltages, the anode's positive potential exerts a weaker attraction on electrons emitted from the filament. As a consequence of this, the residual space charge around the filament tends to be large, representing an unproductive and inefficient emission from the filament. In order to sustain the required rate of electron flow across the tube when operating at low kilovoltages, it is normal practice (space-charge compensation) for the filament temperature to be boosted. There is a limit to the extent to which this can be achieved, however, because higher temperatures increase the rate of vaporization and so threaten to reduce the filament's life.

In a general purpose tube which operates through a kilovoltage range extending up to 120 or 150 kV, a narrowing of the gap between anode and cathode – which would increase mutual attraction – is contra-indicated by the need to maintain electrical safety: to prevent arcing across from one electrode to the other. In mammography tubes, however, which only operate at relatively low kV values, this gap can be narrowed with safety. There is thus no need for highly boosted filament temperatures, to produce given values of tube current.

### Tube mounting

To minimize awkwardness for the patient, the tube housing is made more compact than with a standard, general purpose tube. The technique's relatively low maximum kilovoltage is a favourable factor in allowing the housing to be smaller; and both high tension cables are arranged so that they enter the housing at the anode end, out of the way of the patient's head.

The tube is oriented with the anode further from, and the cathode closer to the patient, to take advantage of the *anode heel effect*. This is rarely significant in general radiography but can usefully be employed in mammography. The intensity of the X-ray beam tends not to be uniform along the tube's axis. From anode to cathode, there is a progressive increase in intensity, as the more open face of the anode appears to the field, implying less absorption of radiation from its source, deep to the surface of the target. Tube mounting is such that the cathode edge of the field exposes the thicker, proximal part of the breast, nearer the chest wall, while the less intense field due to a grazing emission from the anode face is related to the distal part of the breast and the nipple.

### Beam collimation

Beam collimation is consistently accurate, to protect the patient and enhance image contrast, through the rigid link between the X-ray tube and the breast support plate. Since a single technique is being performed, the X-ray beam is collimated by means of a cone which produces a special, D-shaped field.

## 11.3 Compression

Despite assistance from the anode heel effect, the shape of the breast tends to create image density gradients: lighter proximally, darker distally. This variation, which can impede diagnosis, may be lessened by the use of gentle compression. A range of applicators are normally available for mounting on the support which links tube and breast support plate, which incorporate a plastic plate, parallel to the film plane. This can be moved by the radiographer in a carefully controlled manner until it compresses the breast against the support plate. In cases where identified lesions within a breast are being localized or biopsied, the applicator can incorporate a guide to interventional procedures.

Since compression can involve discomfort and anxiety, the mechanism needs to meet two important specifications: gentle, very gradual, controlled application; and immediate, positive release. Hand- or foot-operated controls may be provided.

## 11.4 Exposure timing

Correct image densities are crucial to the diagnostic value of mammographs. Latitude is less than for other radiographic examinations, and students may have observed the stringent quality assurance which surrounds image processing. Quality starts with the accuracy of exposure factors. Variations of breast size and opacity are sufficient, from patient to patient, to make automatic exposure timing an essential feature of mammographic equipment.

The use of low kilovoltages and the breast's relative radiolucency tend to make this more complicated than usual. A D-shaped monitoring area is used. Positioned between breast and film, an ionization chamber may interfere with the image. Positioned behind the film, its reading can be inaccurate, due to absorption and beam quality alteration. A combination of readings with balanced correction is usually employed.

## 11.5  Breast support plate

Aligned accurately to the X-ray beam, and allowing film positioning closely up to the chest wall, a range of plates may be available for use with a range of breast sizes and densities. The supporting surface may be made of carbon fibre which is virtually absorption free. A low ratio grid may be incorporated for use when required.

The lower part of a support plate incorporates lead, to absorb a maximal amount of the primary radiation which otherwise would be transmitted through, to constitute a considerable hazard to the patient's abdomen and pelvis.

## 11.6  Patient reassurance

Handles are provided for the patient to grasp, for steadiness during the procedure, and the manoeuvrability of the equipment can allow the patient to sit, stand or lie down, according to need.

In all situations, the radiographer's skilled psychological care of the patient is all-important. Mammographic units may offer a particular help to the radiographer in demonstrating reassurance, especially to the most nervous and mistrusting patient: the control panel is commonly separated from the patient by a full-length, lead glass protection screen. This enables the radiographer to remain close to the patient during the exposure and clearly at hand to release compression and reassure when an exposure has been completed. The low quality of radiation used for this technique is a favourable factor in allowing this arrangement, while its compact design has enabled mammographic units to be installed in mobile vehicles, to bring the technique – as a screening exercise – into community health settings.

## 11.7  Follow-up practical

The very specialized nature of mammographic work needs to be appreciated before achieving a satisfactory understanding of mammographic equipment.

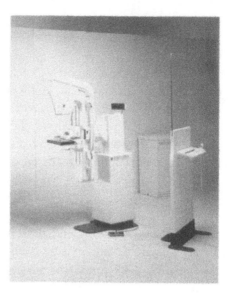

**Fig. 11.3** Mammographic unit. The separate control unit is shown, with its full–height, integral protective screen. This enables the radiographer to stand in safety, close at hand to the patient, while exposures are made. (*By courtesy of IGE Medical Systems.*)

Observe how all the various features of the service relate, one to another, for the benefit of this particular group of patients. Experience should be gained on at least two types of equipment, so that comparative assessments can be made.

# Chapter 12
# Equipment for Conventional Tomography

## 12.1 Introduction

A radiograph is a composite image. Structures lying in the path of the primary X-ray beam cast their shadows on top of each other. Interpretation of this composite is based on being able to distinguish between its component parts, despite the problem of superimposition.

There are situations, however, where superimposition can prevent a diagnosis from being made. A technique is then required which will record an image of the plane or layer of interest on its own, without the obscuring effect of other layers. A radiographic procedure leading to images of selected layers or slices through an object (rather than its whole) is termed **tomography**.

Before the invention of computed tomography, the procedure described here was the only one available. Due to the development of alternative, more reliable techniques, however, its clinical value has declined sharply in recent years. If only in a limited way, however, it is still practised. To avoid ambiguity, it may be known as conventional tomography.

## 12.2 Principle

Separate demonstration of a selected layer through an object is achieved by deliberate movement of X-ray tube and film together, during an exposure. Linkage of tube and film is normally mechanical, by a rigid, metal connecting rod or bar along which, at some point, there is a pivot or fulcrum. Tube and film thus move simultaneously in opposing directions, either along parallel planes or through arcs about a common centre of rotation – the pivot. A unit is currently available, in which there is no physical link between tube and film: instead, computer control ensures their synchronization.

Despite this movement – and possibly contrary to expectations – a sharp image is recorded of the plane through the object, parallel to the film, which passes through the pivot. The sharpness (lack of unsharpness) is due to the fact that there is *no relative movement* between the shadow of this plane and

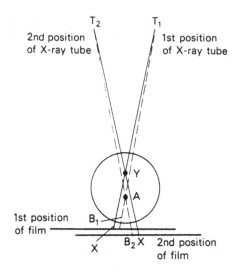

**Fig. 12.1** Principle of tomography. As the X-ray tube moves from $T_1$ to $T_2$, pivoting about Y, the shadow of a structure at Y remains on the film at point X. The shadow of a structure at A moves in relation to the film, from $B_1$ to $B_2$, and so records a blurred impression on the tomographic image. (NB: The film actually stays in the same plane.)

the film: the speed of its shadow exactly matches the speed at which the film travels. This is not true of planes away from the pivot. Their moving shadows either outpace the film or lag behind it during the exposure. This relative movement causes blurring of the effect which such shadows have on the film; it may be debated whether or not they can be described as images. The intention is that they should not be recognizable, whereas the record of the pivot-centred layer is clear. The purpose of tomography is thus achieved: selected structures are shown, free from obscuring overshadowing by others.

## 12.3  Main features of tomographic equipment

The tube–film connecting rod has already been mentioned. It is attached at one end to the tube at the level of the target, and at the other end to the film assembly, at the level of the film itself. The pivot about which tube and film move is housed within a complex unit. Selection of a tomographic layer requires that the pivot must be moveable in relation to the object. It is usual for the pivot to be adjustable along a measuring scale which indicates its position (its *height*) from the table surface on which the patient is supported. The pivot unit also incorporates switches which are responsible for starting and ending the tomographic exposure. This arrangement is quite different from the normal timing of radiographic exposures. Transfer of control from the customary exposure button and timer is due to the need for tomographic exposures to be made only while the tube and film are in motion.

The switches are operated by pressure from the connecting rod, as it moves past. The sequence is as follows:

(1) Pressure on the normal exposure switch (on or attached to the control panel) sets the tube and film off in motion.
(2) Having attained its set speed, the connecting rod approaches and activates the first switch, to start the tomographic exposure.
(3) Tube and film make their planned movements, at constant speed, until the connecting rod reaches the second switch.
(4) The connecting rod's effect on the second switch is to end the tomographic exposure, after which tube and film slow down to a halt.

It is clear, therefore, that these switches have considerable importance. This is enhanced by the fact that they are adjustable: they can be moved to alter the exposure time and, more significantly, the exposure angle. Calibration of the switches' positions is actually shown in terms of exposure angle, more often than as exposure time.

From repeated mention of movement, it is clear that some form of drive is required. This is an electric motor, usually with the option of speed variation, to enable exposure time to be controlled other than by switch position.

## Tomographic layer thickness

Mention has been made of the *height* or position of the tomographic layer within the object. This, naturally, is adjusted according to the anatomical structure being examined. For example, if a supine patient is being tomographed, a posterior structure will require a relatively low pivot position, while a more anterior structure will be shown by raising the pivot to a higher position.

No mention has yet been made, however, of the thickness of the tomographic layer: how much of the object is recorded on the image? The answer depends on how effectively the shadows of structures lying on either side of the pivot plane have been blurred. If completely blurred and unrecognizable, the tomographic layers which remain sharp will be thin. If only slightly blurred and still mostly recognizable, the structures represented by these shadows will remain as parts within a relatively thick layer.

The three principal factors affecting layer thickness will be discussed.

### The exposure angle

Adjustment of the exposure switches increases or reduces the distances travelled by tube and film (their excursions). It will be remembered that movement is responsible for the tomographic effect. It follows that the greater this movement and the unsharpness it causes, the narrower will be the layer recorded as a sharp tomographic image. Conversely, slight movement, through a small angle, will allow structures remote from the pivot plane to form sharp images and remain within a relatively thick layer.

### Tomographic trajectory (pattern of tube/film movement)

Recognizability of blurred structures will depend on whether movement has been simply along a straight line, in which case there will be linear blurring, possibly failing to disguise the shadows' origins, or whether movement has been more complex – circular, for example – which is much more likely to blur shadows beyond recognition.

### The shape of the structure being tomographed

Ideally, there should be little correlation between tomographic trajectory and object shape. A linear object will tend to be shown better by a linear trajectory if it lies transversely across the object's axis than if it aligns to this axis. Results may be better still with an unrelated, more complex trajectory. These factors have implications for the equipment used for tomography – for the facilities and limitations of the types available.

## 12.4  Types of tomographic equipment

Students will encounter two categories: tomographic attachments to convert basic radiographic equipment (tube and couch); and specialized, dedicated tomographic units.

### *Tomographic attachments*

An attachment comprises three parts: the connecting rod, pivot unit and drive unit with its controls. The connecting rod is made to attach to the X-ray tube along the transverse axis of its mount. With the rotation brake released, allowing beam angulation along the couch, the connecting rod links tube movement parallel to the couch with movement of the bucky assembly along its rails beneath the couch top. A feature of the connecting rod is that it must be extendable in length, either by having a telescopic construction or by making a sliding connection to either the tube or film mount. This arrangement then accommodates the change in focus–film distance which occurs during the tube/film excursion. At the start of the exposure and when it ends, the focus–film distance is greater than during the exposure. At the midpoint, when the tube is directing its beam at right-angles to the film, the focus–film distance is at its minimum.

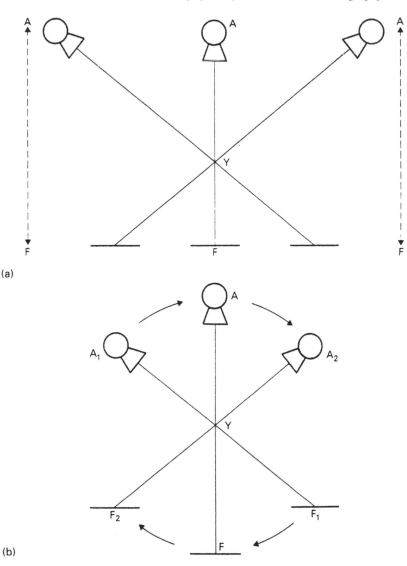

**Fig. 12.2** Tomographic movements. (a) Line-to-line movement is produced by a tomographic attachment: vertical height of the tube is fixed, and the focus–film distance is variable. (b) The arc-to-arc movement offered by a specialized unit maintains a constant focus–film distance.

Attachment to the pivot unit is typically via a sliding groove, to allow for focus–film distance extension and shortening during the exposure. The pivot unit fixes to one of the couch's side rails. Its pivot can be adjusted up and down a scale which indicates height above the couch top. Widening and narrowing of the gap between the exposure switches alters the exposure angle. Adjustment may be symmetrical or allow individual variations on either side of the midline.

An electric drive unit may already form part of the tube mount. In this case, the tomographic attachment forms an amendment to its controls, transferring switching to the exposure circuitry and providing a speed adjustment facility.

An attachment is the least expensive form of tomographic equipment and it allows the X-ray tube and couch to operate with their full versatility, when it is not in place. In an imaging department where tomography is a rarely requested procedure, its facilities may be sufficient to meet this need. Tomographic attachments have their limitations, however. Only a long-itudinal linear trajectory is offered. As has been mentioned, this may not be suitable for some anatomical subjects. The parallel plane tube/film excursions, with varying focus–film distance, tend to bias image densities towards the central parts of the exposure, rather than providing an even image density formation. Assembling and connecting the attachment takes time and, with prolonged use, introduces mechanical slackness and inaccuracy.

In summary, image quality may not reach the highest value.

### Specialized tomographic units

With the decline in popularity of conventional tomography, these units have become more or less obsolete. Relatively high expense and limited facilities for performing other radiographic procedures have contributed to this. For tomographic images of the highest quality, however, their use continues to provide useful service, where the clinical demand is retained. Quality arises from the range of multi-directional trajectories available, mechanical integrity and accuracy, and refinement of controls.

Convenience comes from permanent assembly – they are always ready for use. Complex gearing provides a range of trajectories which may include transverse as well as longitudinal linear, circular, elliptical, spiral, hypocy-cloidal (*trefoil*) and lissajous (*figure-of-eight*). Together these can match all anatomical shape requirements and, by angular variation, allow wide ranges of layer thicknesses to be produced. Instead of having parallel plane trajectories, tube and film may both move through arcs, centred on the pivot. As well as being mechanically smoother, this arrangement maintains a constant focus–film distance during the exposure. Pivot adjustment may be achieved by raising and lowering the patient on a variable height couch top. This brings the advantage of constant magnification for all images.

A specialized unit may also provide facilities for simultaneous multi-section tomography. This technique, using a deep cassette, containing typically three or five sets of intensifying screens and films, separated by measured spacers, offers the theoretical advantage of achieving three or five tomographs (of spaced layers) simultaneously with a single exposure – with all the radiation protection and time-saving benefits arising from this

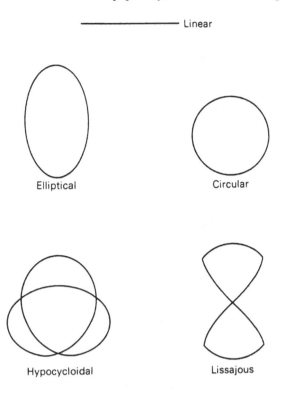

Fig. 12.3 Tomographic trajectories. The more complicated, multi-directional trajectories achieve a less recognizable impression of structures remote from the fulcrum layer, but imply lengthened exposure times, compared with a simple linear trajectory.

economy. In practice, however, there are obstacles to achieving equality of image definition which bring the technique's validity into question.

Equipment is available which strikes a balance between the truly and exclusively *dedicated* on the one hand, and the attachment option, on the other. Tomographic facilities are commonly available as an option on equipment in which the tube and the bucky/cassette assembly are permanently linked. Smooth, synchronized movement – even though the movement may be restricted to longitudinal linear – can produce very adequate tomographs, when the need arises.

## 12.5 Equipment tests

Wherever mechanical equipment is involved, there is a need periodically to check that *wear and tear* are not reducing function and efficiency. This rule applies to tomographic equipment no less than to other machines. There is a problem here, however. Tomographic images, formed by movement, and

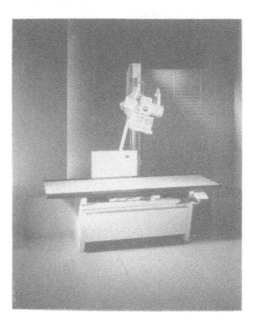

**Fig. 12.4** An integrated radiographic unit with tomographic facilities. This type of unit is becoming popular because of its versatility. The X-ray tube is linked to the central bucky assembly by a connection which can instantly allow tomography to be performed, when required. The mechanical weaknesses of an add-on attachment are eliminated and the unit can be used for all routine radiographic techniques. (*By courtesy of IGE Medical Systems.*)

varying according to anatomical and pathological conditions, give no clear, definite sign of mechanical malfunction. Image deficiencies can arise from other sources – a fact which has probably contributed to the technique's declining popularity.

Tomographic tests therefore tend to be carried out on little used equipment, in no real expectation of discovering an abnormality. Their perpetuation – among students, at least – is largely due to their simplicity and satisfyingly clear results. Commercial test equipment is available but otherwise, *home-made* equipment can function well, particularly to test linear equipment, to show:

(1) Accuracy of pivot height – is it exactly as shown on the scale or has mechanical wear made the pivot loose and imprecise?
(2) Integrity of movement – do film and tube move exactly along their planned trajectories or is there some vibration which causes deviation?
(3) Accuracy of exposure angle – do the exposure switches start and end the exposure, exactly as set?

A further test procedure is valuable, not as a check on the equipment's

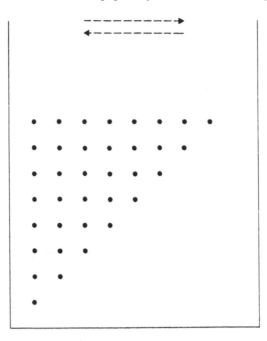

**Fig. 12.5** A simple phantom for checking tomographic pivot height. Metal pins inserted into the side of a wooden or plastic block show vertical heights in centimetres above the base (in contact with the couch top). A linear tomograph will demonstrate sharp images of pins which lie at the pivot height; these should number the height in centimetres.

accuracy but with the important aim of measuring the thickness of tomographic layer produced by different trajectories and exposure angles. The information gained from this investigation is invaluable as a guide to the correct employment of tomographic procedures when there is a clinical indication that they are needed.

## 12.6 Follow-up practical

(1) Find your clinical department's tomographic equipment, even if this means seeking out and assembling attachments which have not been used for a long time. Explore its practical operation. If possible, make comparisons between the facilities provided by different units, particularly those which are *dedicated*.

(2) Investigative procedures should be performed on both constructed (metal, plastic) and anatomical phantoms, to discover tomographic capabilities and limitations.

(3) Carry out tests for the accuracy of pivot height, exposure angle settings and movement integrity, using the test equipment available.

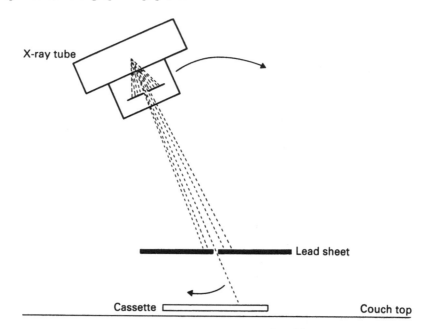

**Fig. 12.6** Principle of a test for integrity of tomographic movement. A stationary film positioned on the couch top is exposed to a narrow, pencil beam of X-rays transmitted through a small hole in a lead sheet, supported above and parallel to the film. A tomographic exposure is made and, while the tube moves through its tomographic trajectory, the transmitted X-ray beam sweeps through a reciprocal pattern below the lead sheet. Momentary slowing or deviation of movement produces darker areas or irregularity of the traced image.

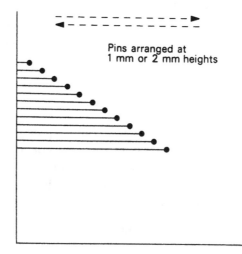

**Fig. 12.7** A simple phantom to measure tomographic layer thickness. This phantom can be used with a linear trajectory. Pins inserted in the vertical face of a wooden or plastic box mark the boundaries of the layer by recording sharp images on the test tomograph. For example, three sharp images of pins at 1 mm intervals indicate a thickness of approximately 2 mm.

# Part Six
# Computer-Based Imaging Modalities

A student radiographer's earliest practical experience of imaging involves projection of an X-ray beam through the patient's body, from an X-ray tube on one side to a film or screen on the other. Images are thus formed simply and directly by transmitted X-ray shadows.

The final part of this text covers equipment concerned with creating diagnostic images by methods more complicated than simple X-ray transmission.

Since, increasingly, image construction methods are employing the facilities offered by computers, and because computers handle data fed to them in digital form, Chapter 13 outlines the principles of image digitization.

An X-ray tube is still the imaging energy source in computed tomography, although here the transmitted X-ray beam exposes detectors, rather than a screen or film. Computed tomography equipment is described in Chapter 14.

The last three chapters of this text cover imaging modalities far removed from radiography or fluoroscopy. Radionuclide imaging (Chapter 15) concerns the conversion into an image, of radiation which emanates from the patient's body. Medical ultrasound images are formed when energy (significantly, non-ionizing) emitted by the equipment is reflected back along its original path (Chapter 16); while magnetic resonance imaging equipment controls a complex sequence of emission and detection, as described in Chapter 17.

# Chapter 13
# Image Digitization

## 13.1 Introduction

**Digitization** is a term becoming widely used in several fields – perhaps most commonly in home entertainment. We are becoming familiar with **digital** recordings, for example. This chapter attempts to outline the principle of image digitization, explain some of its potential benefits and describe their radiographic applications.

## 13.2 The difference between analogue and digital

The alternative to digital is **analogue,** a word which, to some extent, has been rediscovered to describe the ordinary or natural. The two terms commonly appear as descriptions of contrasting types of clocks and watches. The old-fashioned type with hands sweeping across a face gives a smooth, continuously changing analogue display. Digital displays are arguably easier to read – or, at least, more difficult to misread. To extend the time analogy: human civilization has subdivided the day into units: hours, minutes and seconds. Thus, while in fact the earth spins smoothly on its axis, there is a convenience in having subdivisions as points of reference, for measurement and identification.

### Sampling

An analogue signal is converted into a digital signal via a process of regular, periodic measurement, termed **sampling**. For accuracy, the frequency of sampling is all-important. A relatively low sampling rate results in a coarse digital signal which may fail to preserve sudden or subtle variations in the original analogue. The example of time measurement may provide an illustration on this point. A digital clock which records and displays minutes could be used satisfactorily for timing a football match. The more frequent time sampling display of hundredths of a second would be essential for timing a sprint race. A simple rule may govern choice of sampling rate: a balance between need and expense.

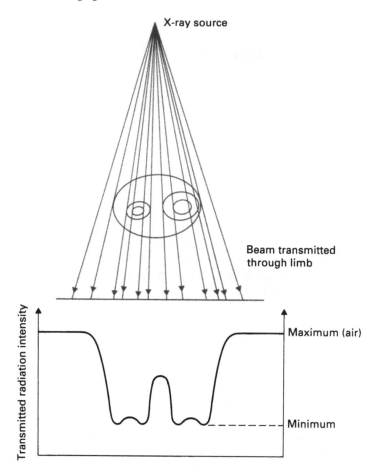

**Fig. 13.1** Analogue signal formation from transmitted X-rays. Due to the naturally rounded shape of body structures, there tends to be an absence of sudden change.

### Creation of an image signal

The principle needs to be addressed of converting an image such as a radiograph, which occupies an area, into a simple, continuous signal. Basically, scanning is used, as in a television or a fax machine, where an image is converted into a signal for transmission from one place to another via a telephone line or radio waves.

The formation of a digital image requires the signal obtained from scanning to be digitized. For this purpose it is scanned – a procedure which divides the image up into fine, narrow horizontal rows, and during which the scanning point takes measurements or samples at fine, regular intervals. Samples taken at the same position along successive rows form vertical columns, at 90° to the rows. A digital image can thus be thought of as being marked out like graph paper into a matrix of squares. The squares are called

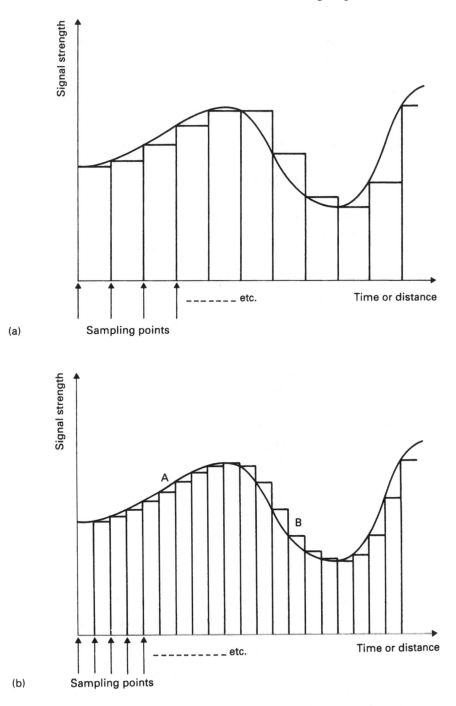

**Fig. 13.2** Analogue to digital conversion. (a) Coarse sampling of an analogue signal. (b) More frequent sampling. A reduction in the sampling interval brings the profile of the digital signal closer to the analogue. Sampling rate is more critical when the signal variation is more marked. Compare gradients A and B.

**pixels** (an abbreviation of picture elements). Each has a set of co-ordinates indicating its precise position (termed its **address**) within the matrix image, in a row and a column. Each pixel is thus individually identifiable. Its address contains numerical information about signal strength in that location.

## 13.3  The benefits of diagnostic image digitization

Computed tomography and magnetic resonance imaging are modalities in which images are constructed from gathered image data which is already in digital form. Ultrasound and radionuclide imaging are employing digitization more prominently and its introduction into fluoroscopy, in specialized angiographic techniques, is now being followed by an application to radiography. A radiographic image recorded on film with the aid of intensifying screens, or on the output screen of an image intensifier, can be scanned by a high resolution television camera whose output video signal is then digitized. High resolution TV systems at present operate on 1250 lines. To give optimum results, vertical and horizontal resolution should match, i.e. the matrix should be symmetrically based.

To be acceptable as a replacement for a conventional radiographic image on film, a digital system must offer an equal standard of resolution, unless it is acceptable that some information, in certain circumstances, is not essential for an accurate diagnosis. Poor spatial resolution will not distinguish between adjacent objects, but high resolution equipment is expensive. In practice, a compromise is reached, with sampling occurring at a frequency which will ensure that the required image detail is demonstrated. The important question in any situation is what resolution is needed for an accurate and reliable diagnosis.

To achieve acceptable results in most situations, a radiograph would need to be sampled at least every 0.2 mm, giving a maximum theoretical resolution of 2.5 line pairs (one black and one white stripe) per mm, recorded in adjacent pixels. The pixels also need to be able to record grey levels, of which there are typically 1024 (10 bit). The significance of the 10 bit is that it is a binary number, thus something which computers can handle easily.

As an alternative to film or an image intensifier, a special imaging plate may be used: exposure to X-rays creating electronic changes (akin to formation of the latent image in a film emulsion) which are then read by a high resolution laser scanner. This signal is then digitized, either for display on a monitor or as a hard copy. The resolution available from a laser reader is far better than anything of which the imaging plate is capable, so there is no risk of information being lost. In theory, the user could (as above) decide

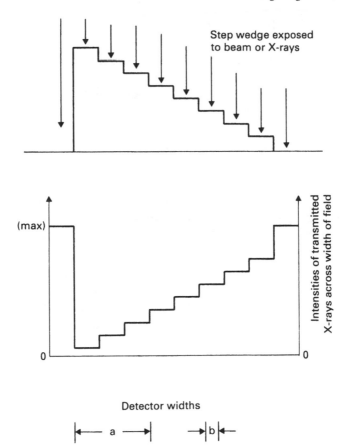

**Fig. 13.3** Detector width. In any given situation, when a digital signal is formed, the detectors must be small enough and placed sufficiently close together for reliable point measurements. In the above example, a detector of width a will be unable to distinguish between (resolve) individual steps of the wedge. The narrower detector, b, will be able to resolve individual steps but adjacent measurements may be variable in their alignment with step boundaries. Reliability is achieved in practice by frequently repeated sampling (e.g. many times per cycle).

upon the resolution required, up to a maximum. There is no doubt that the importance of this system will continue to increase.

The conversion of an analogue image into an image made up of squares is not the complete story, however. Especially in view of the enduring, widespread use of film and intensifying screens, the expense and complication of digitizing radiographic images would seem to be in need of some justification.

An X-ray film may be identified as having three roles. Satisfaction of these explains its long-standing use but, also, its shortcomings support the argument for change. To some extent, the fact that film has three roles also explains the complications associated with any replacement system.

The three functions of an X-ray film are as follows:

(1) It is a **detector**: its emulsions are sensitive to image-forming energies.

This property is not unique: fluorescent and electrically-charged screens can also detect radiation *images*.

(2) When processed, an exposed film becomes a radiographic image **display**.

The speed and neatness of this transition, brought about by chemical processing, is a convenience and a strong advantage. Unfortunately, it is also a restriction. The displayed information cannot substantially be changed. For example, a postero-anterior radiograph of the lung fields remains just that. Although the patient's thoracic vertebrae also lie within the irradiated area, it requires a separate, additional exposure to display them.

Digitization of a signal derived from an image allows many options in the manner of displaying the detected image information.

(3) A radiograph is a **storage** device: its information is retained for future reference.

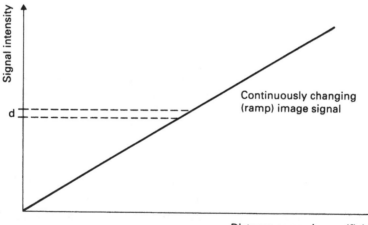

Fig. 13.4 Digitized contrast detection. A continuous gradient or ramp can be considered to have an infinite number of steps between its top and bottom. If two narrowly differing signal intensities, separated by difference d, are displayed conventionally on film, the eye may be unable to distinguish between them. If the signal is digitized, however (effectively reducing the number of steps), small differences such as d can be exaggerated and displayed. In practice, many more step readings (*levels of grey*) are taken than can be displayed, so that a selective display (a *window*) needs to be chosen, according to the imaged feature requirements.

Again, there are advantages and limitations. To be able to open up an envelope and withdraw a radiograph, immediately ready for viewing, is an undoubted convenience. To have to transport it physically between departments or from hospital to hospital, without loss or damage, is a practical limitation. To have to find space for its long-term storage is a problem which, in some hospitals, becomes a nightmare.

A digitized image can be stored in a computer memory, in a compact form which is unrivalled. Imaging departments are already being created which are virtually *filmless*. Access to this information, its immediate display on high resolution monitors and, indeed, its transmission across the world is a relatively simple task. Its combination with digitized data from other sources is another valuable facility.

The increasing application of image digitization to diagnostic imaging modalities is largely due to the opportunities provided for image manipulation, essential to which is the assigning of numerical values to the samples recorded in each pixel's address (once it is understood what these numbers refer to).

## Windowing

The digital output as displayed on a TV monitor shows a linear response, unlike film which has a characteristic curve. The digital TV display is said to have a greater dynamic range. This also means that its tolerance to over-exposure is greater than film's – a point which needs to be carefully monitored, to ensure that radiation dose levels to the patient are not exceeding an acceptable level. In fact the range of image densities acquired and stored is too great, both for the display to cope with and for the eye to appreciate. Rather than being a problem, this is a distinct advantage because it allows users to select the image density (signal) range in which they are interested. This range selection – a commonly practised form of manipulation – is termed windowing.

The window can be moved up or down the range of densities available, to establish a window height or level; and its size can be varied (window width selection) so that image contrast can be varied, i.e. the range of actual densities represented within a given image. Window level selection is well illustrated in computed tomography where, from a single set of data (single exposure to the patient) the image can display any level through from soft tissue to skeletal details.

Once an image is in digital form, a whole range of other manipulations can be performed: images can be enhanced and highlighted (possibly with colour); and new images can be reconstructed from selected data originally acquired for different purposes.

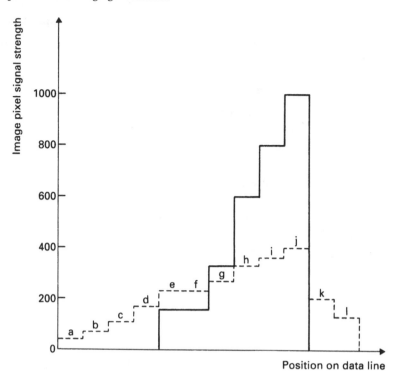

**Fig. 13.5** Contrast improvement. The broken line shows a measured (raw data) signal strength variation, with limited contrast between e and j. Computer manipulation of these values can increase the contrast, as shown by the solid line. A 200–400 width was set, all values below 200 being suppressed. The readings between 200 and 400 were scaled up to a 0–1000 range.

## 13.4 Follow-up practical

The commonest imaging modalities presently available, which demonstrate these manipulation options, are computed tomography and digital fluoroscopy. Request a demonstration from the clinical staff who operate this equipment, so that its versatility can be appreciated first-hand.

# Chapter 14
# Computed Tomography

## 14.1 Introduction

Computed tomography (commonly abbreviated to CT) is a procedure which creates images of sections through the the patient's body. On this account, it is termed **tomography**. Students who have previous experience only of conventional X-ray tomography should recognize that any attempt at comparison between these two procedures would be unsuccessful and potentially confusing. They are similar in name only. Computed tomography images are created by a computer from digitized data obtained by exposing the patient to X-rays in a particular manner. The computer is able to manipulate data so that, from a single X-ray exposure, many different images can be obtained, using the facilities which the combination of digitization and specialized software (computer programs) can provide.

## 14.2 The principle of CT

The X-ray tube is fitted with a collimating device which confines its emission to a very narrow, flat, *fan* beam, covering an angle of between 30 and 50°. The beam is accurately aligned to an array of small radiation detectors in the form of an arc, each equidistant from the X-ray tube's focal spot. In front of each detector is a collimator which limits its measurement to the rays approaching that detector along a line from the focal spot. The detectors are able accurately to measure X-ray intensity. These measurements are digitized and fed to a computer.

If the beam is attenuated, the detectors' measurements can be translated to indicate the amount of attenuation which has occurred (from the difference between the two intensity measurements – direct and with attenuation). These attenuation measurements can be translated into data indicating the relative opacities of structures lying in the path of the X-ray beam, between the focal spot and each detector.

If a patient's body (part) is positioned in the path of this narrow, fan beam, with both tube and detectors in fixed, static positions, the array of detectors effectively divides up a thin section of the body into linear strips.

Each detector measures the X-ray attenuation which has occurred within, and thus the opacity of, its own aligned strip of this section. If this information were to be displayed on the computer's monitor screen, it would appear as a very thin strip of a radiographic image. This exercise would serve no purpose; it would lack an essential feature: movement.

During CT, the X-ray tube rotates around the patient's body, making exposures at different angles, as it moves along its circular path. On the opposite side of the body, the detectors are measuring the attenuation occurring within the narrow strips of the body to which they are aligned. The data obtained from the sequence of measured transmissions constitute an absorption profile or projection. A movement of the equipment round the patient is described as rotation. These measurement signals are digitized and stored in the computer's memory.

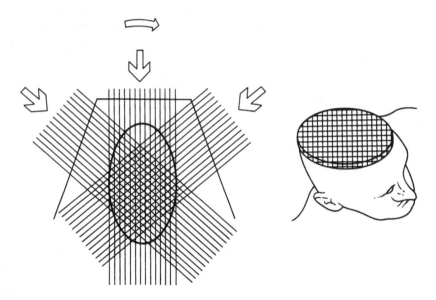

Fig. 14.1 Creation of a matrix. Exposures at angular intervals, received by an array of detectors, create a matrix in a transverse plane.

At the end of the CT exposure, when the X-ray tube has completed its movement, the computer has stored information about the opacities of strips through the body, created at all the different angles at which exposures have been made. The effect of the rotation, as the X-rays have criss-crossed the body section, has been to create small, discrete areas rather than strips. These are actually small *volumes*: their dimensions determined by the thickness (narrowness) of the X-ray beam, the width of individual detectors and the number of angles from which measurements are made, during the exposure. They are termed **voxels**, a word formed from volume elements.

The computer thus has information in its memory about the X-ray attenuation which has occurred within the thousands of strips through the body, measured at all the various angles. It is now able very quickly to perform calculations which result in measurement of the relative opacities (indicating composition and tissue type) of each individual voxel. These readings are then translated into image brightness levels and displayed on its monitor screen. Each voxel is represented in two-dimensional form as a picture element cell, termed a **pixel**.

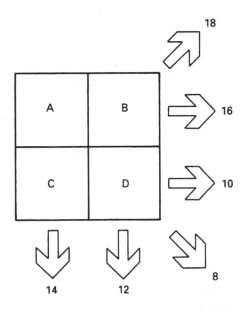

**Fig. 14.2** Exercise to illustrate calculation of attenuation values from aggregate transmission data. In this 2 × 2 matrix, the values of A, B, C and D can be calculated from the sums measured along horizontal, vertical and diagonal axes. For example:

$B + A = 16$
$B + C = 18$
Therefore $C = A + 2$
But $A + C = 14$
Therefore $A = 6$ and $C = 8$

In a similar manner, the CT computer calculates attenuation values for the voxels within the matrix created by alignment of the detectors which measure transmitted X-ray intensities. Note that the measurements (sums/transmitted intensities) exceed the minimum required for calculation. These additional measurements are used to check the accuracy of the calculations ($B = 10$ and $D = 2$).

The number of pixels within a CT image (depending on detector size and distribution, and exposure frequency) determines the resolution with which the section through the object is portrayed. There is usually a 512 × 512 matrix, in which there are approximately 260 000 voxels/pixels.

When the X-ray beam passes through the body, it is traversing a succession of volumes of different kinds of tissue. Depending upon the nature of its composition, each successive volume may differently reduce the incident intensity. Thus, the X-ray intensity of the beam at an exit point is the sum of a series of fractionations of the beam which have occurred within the irradiated volume. If the internal structure of that volume is to be accurately determined, in order to create a detailed image of it, the various fractionations of the incident beam must be evaluated separately. That is, an absorption value must be computed for each separate *block* within the irradiated material. Then, one tissue can be differentiated from another.

Digitization of the emergent X-ray intensities involves assigning to each pixel a number which represents the attenuation occurring within the corresponding voxel. These are calculated mathematically by the computer. A number of mathematical methods (in computer language: algorithms) are available, any of which should yield the data required for image construction. Each provides the computer with a coherent approach to solving the problem. Its ultimate purpose is to bring the pixels to their simplest ratios so that an image of faithfully related densities can be constructed.

## 14.3 Equipment for CT

Every CT equipment unit (normally referred to as a **scanner** since it originally entered the clinical field, following the pioneering work of Sir Godfrey Hounsfield, as *EMI-scanning*; it is basically a scanning technique) comprises the following parts:

(1) A **gantry** or frame which incorporates the X-ray tube, beam collimating equipment and the detectors which measure radiation intensity. Centrally, there is a circular or elliptical aperture within which the patient is positioned.

(2) An X-ray **generator**, supplying energy to the X-ray tube.

(3) A **table** on which the patient lies, capable of being very accurately positioned with respect to the X-ray beam, and equipped with finely controllable motor drives.

(4) An operator's **console** from where all the various complex functions can be selected and monitored.

(5) A **computer** which receives the X-ray intensity signals and is programmed to provide the resources necessary for their interpretation, manipulation and display as CT images.

(6) A computer **memory** storage/recall facility.

(7) A **hard copy** unit.

This equipment is housed in a room which, more particularly than other radiodiagnostic rooms, has a stabilized temperature and relative humidity. This is important for the computer's reliable operation, under conditions specified by the equipment manufacturer, free from the risk of overheating and condensation.

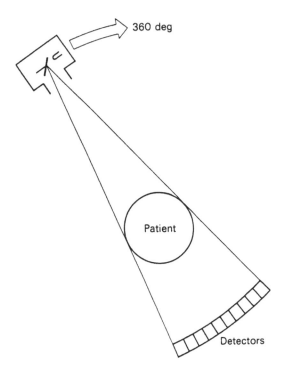

360 deg

Patient

Detectors

**Fig. 14.3** CT: X-ray tube aligned to and rotating with a limited arc of detectors.

## *The scanning gantry*

Since it was originally conceived, a CT scanner has undergone a number of radical changes, termed *generations*. Each change has been intended to increase the scanner's efficiency and safety, and the quality of its images.

The central aperture through which the patient lies needs to be able to accommodate a large adult abdomen. If the aperture is too large, image quality suffers; if too small, there is a risk of not being able to accept some patients, while others may experience claustrophobia. Careful design may combat this last effect by making the aperture appear larger than it really is.

If the gantry plane is at right-angles to the table, CT images will show normal transverse planes through the body (supine). For some purposes, however, oblique planes may align more exactly with the anatomical structures which are being examined. In some instances, the patient's position may be adapted, so that an oblique plane is presented to the normal path of the X-ray beam. Otherwise, this relationship can be achieved more

safely and comfortably if it is possible to tilt the whole gantry up to 20°
cranio–caudad from its vertical position. The provision of this facility will
require an increase in the dimensions of the aperture. Oblique angulation of
the table (still in a horizontal plane) termed **slewing** can also affect the
aperture design.

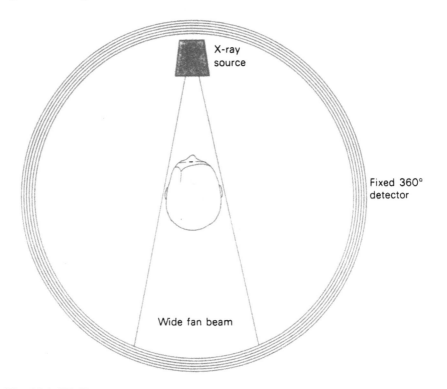

Fig. 14.4 CT: X-ray tube moving independently within a fixed ring of detectors.

### The X-ray tube

A heavy duty rotating anode tube is required, with a high anode thermal
capacity. This may be achieved by the use of a conventional tube with a
thick graphite backing to the compound metallic disc, to raise its thermal
capacity to over a million joules without proportionately increasing its
weight; or a metal–ceramic tube with a large diameter anode disc supported
on a through axle, mounted at both ends. As well as requiring a very high
thermal capacity, the focal spot size needs to be small, to maintain the
geometric definition of the image; it may typically be 0.5 mm. The maximum ratio between true and effective focal areas can be achieved by use of
an anode disc with a flat front surface. The radiation emitted in the direction
of the tube window is thus the tangential fraction confined by the disc itself.

In current clinical practice, there are two alternative arrangements of tube
and radiation detectors:

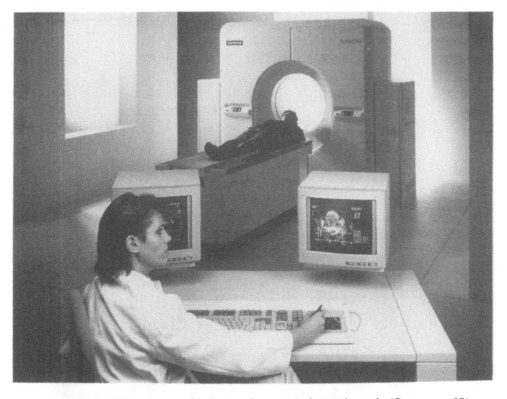

**Fig. 14.5** CT equipment, showing couch, gantry and control console. (*By courtesy of Siemens plc.*)

**(1)** The X-ray tube may be rigidly coupled to an arc of detectors which are precisely aligned and confined to the X-ray beam. Tube and detector array move together around a fixed point in space, at the centre of the gantry's aperture, i.e. the centre of the anatomical subject. Radiation output from the tube is pulsed, as rotation proceeds, to achieve a succession of angular projections.

**(2)** The X-ray tube may be independently moveable through a circular path, with its fan beam aligned to a limited arc within a complete, permanently fixed ring of detectors. Movement of the tube around its circular path continuously changes the particular arc of detectors to which the beam is aligned, while exposure is continuous. This arrangement simplifies the mechanical provision for movement. It also has its drawbacks, however:

(a) Having a large number of detectors increases its price, both for purchase and maintenance.

(b) Its geometry tends to be poor: to allow room for passage of the X-ray tube, a space is necessary between the patient and the detectors. This

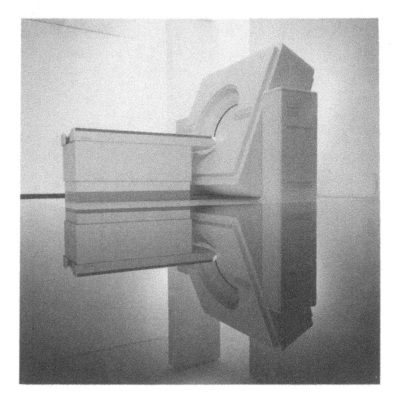

**Fig. 14.6** CT gantry in tilted position. This angulation facility enables an oblique plane through the head or body to be imaged directly. (*By courtesy of Siemens plc.*)

allows for spread of penumbra, thus limiting spatial resolution, and inherently increasing magnification.

(c) Its cost effectiveness may be questioned, since only a limited number of its detectors are receiving radiation, at any given time.

Tube and detector movements are motor driven, to achieve accuracy, smoothness and speed. While short exposure times are important to eliminate patient movement and the image artefacts this can produce, there are problems inherent in fast systems. When photons are few, due to their random arrival at the detectors, the image is subject to increased **noise** (akin to the quantum mottle which may affect radiographs). Because of this limitation, fast scanners may have to run at less than their maximum speeds, if images of the highest diagnostic quality are to be produced.

If each detector is focused on the X-ray source (like the radiolucent spaces of a focused secondary radiation grid) less scattered radiation is received. When detectors are inefficient in rejecting scatter, the sensitivity of the system to contrast is reduced and density discrimination impaired. It would be a feature of the ideal scanner that the detectors were subject to no scattered radiation: in practice this cannot be realized. Scanning systems are therefore designed to ensure that the acceptance of scatter is as low as possible.

Other critical factors are the spacing between detectors and detector aperture size. Close packing together of a relatively large number of detectors in an array is the ideal for all emergent X-ray photons to contribute to the image. A small detector aperture size increases spatial resolution and assists in low acceptance of scatter. It also reduces dose efficiency, however, because some unscattered, emergent X-rays are undetected.

Performance criteria of a detector are:

(1) Having a good detection efficiency. This term refers to its ability to absorb X-ray photon energy. Not only do undetected photons fail to contribute to the image data, they needlessly increase the radiation dose received by the patient.
(2) Having a wide dynamic range. This term refers to a detector's ability to receive a wide range of X-ray intensities, from low to high, and convert them into proportional output signals. If beam intensity exceeds the dynamic range, errors occur in the acquisition of radiation data and the images are marred by artefacts.

Radiation detectors used in CT scanners may be either crystal scintillation detectors, working in conjunction with photomultipliers, or gas ionization detectors.

### Crystal detectors

These may be crystals of sodium iodide, caesium iodide or bismuth germinate. Coupled with each crystal is a photomultiplier which detects the emitted light and converts it into an amplified electrical signal. Close detector spacing may require a smaller device, a photodiode, to be used. This is simpler and smaller than a photomultiplier but produces a weaker signal, requiring a higher degree of amplification which can allow an increase in image noise.

The detection efficiency of a *good* crystal generally is higher than the same property of a detector which depends on the ionization of a gas; but a crystal array may be less stable in the long term, due to lack of uniformity in the crystal's response, persistence of light emission after irradiation has ceased (afterglow) and ageing.

### Gas ionization detectors

These contain the inert gas, xenon. Detection efficiency is relatively low in comparison with scintillation crystal detectors. The gas is maintained at high pressure to increase detection efficiency, and heighten uniformity of response to exposure.

Advantages of a xenon detector system include: constant sensitivity in both short and long terms; indifference to changes in ambient temperature and humidity; wide dynamic range; and rapid response, without afterglow. The relatively small size favours use in the construction of large detector arrays.

## 14.4 The X-ray generator

To maximize imaging efficiency, a constant potential supply is required; the kilovoltage must be stable, since fluctuation tends to cause image artefacts. Three-phase, 12-pulse, middle or high frequency outputs satisfy this need. Typically an output range of 100 to 150 kV is required.

## 14.5 The table

The table supports the patient. It is motor driven to provide finely controlled (millimetre at a time) height adjustment and horizontal movement through and within the gantry aperture, so that any selected section may be examined. Location and centring are indicated by a laser beam coupled with a digital display. Controls for positioning the patient are incorporated into or located adjacent to the table. Horizontal table movement can also be initiated from the operator's console actually during an exposure. Movement while the tube and detectors are stationary produces an image termed a **topogram**. This may resemble a plain radiograph – of the thorax or abdomen, for example – but it is different in lacking the distortion which beam divergence tends to cause. It also bears calibrated reference data to aid its use in selecting appropriate centring for subsequent CT images.

In most situations, CT equipment is not very adaptable to patients' needs; it is they who must adapt to the equipment. Slewing, however, together with gantry tilting, may allow standardized images to be obtained when patients are comatose, injured or paralysed with awkward deformity of the body, without causing distress.

## 14.6 The operating/display console

The console provides push button control of the numerous functions, from the simple – mechanical movement of the patient, and initiating an exposure – through to the complex computer controls and image filing and recall commands. There is a keyboard for the input of patient identification data (name, date, scan parameters, etc.) and for communication with the computer, and a monitor screen for viewing the images, in black and white or in colour.

## 14.7 The computer

The computer receives large quantities of digitized, raw data derived from the transmitted X-ray intensities measured by the detectors. Calculations are performed at high speed, to yield attenuation data relating to each voxel within the irradiated section through the object and each pixel in the CT image. Typically, matrixes might be $512 \times 512$, yielding over 260 000 pixels for one image – and proof of the necessity for a large computer memory.

In their raw state, the differences between data relating to adjacent voxels/pixels may be quite small and difficult to appreciate, especially if overall there is a wide range from minimum to maximum values. A scan of the chest, for instance, may yield values ranging from that relating to air within the lungs to the signal generated by the densest part of the thoracic skeleton.

In practice, therefore, in order more usefully to display such attenuation differences, a conversion factor is applied. This magnifies all the numbers but, importantly, also magnifies the differences between them. The outcome of this process is a series of values for the image pixels, termed CT numbers.

CT numbers are not absolute for any particular tissue. They vary with photon energy. This is bound to be so, since they involve absorption processes. As in more familiar instances of exposure to X-rays (in diagnostic radiography), attenuation coefficients are a function of the beam quality; so, as kilovoltage increases, coefficients tend to reduce. Thus CT numbers will tend to vary between different CT equipment units, depending upon the kilovoltage and filtration of the X-ray beam.

Television monitors offer a suitable means of displaying the signals from the voxels: CT numbers, with their varying values, are translated into various shades of grey on a black-and-white monitor (or into colours for display on a colour monitor).

There is, however, an incompatibility between the 15 to 20 shades of grey recognizable on a television monitor and the very great range of attenuation values acquired by the scanner. To meet this discrepancy, scanners use a **windowing** system. This refers to the selection at any one time of only a group of CT numbers from within the large range.

Push button selection at the console allows the scanner's operator to select a width of window (marked by chosen minimum and maximum values) from within the whole range; and a level of the window, that is, the position of the selected window within the whole available scale. Information about the window – its selected width, its upper limit, centre and lower limit – should be included on each image, for reference, alongside the alphanumeric data relating to patient identification.

Density values (representing attenuation values) reproduce white on the monitor screen when they lie above the window limit and black when they lie below the window limit, giving a continuous grey scale of CT numbers *enclosed* within the window.

A windowing technique during visualization of a CT image, as described, is one of the several data manipulations which are possible, for modifying the image at will, in order to obtain specific information. This is one of the assets of image digitization which has made CT so important as a clinical technique.

Other data manipulation techniques are available, depending mainly upon the **software** (operating programs) with which the computer is equipped. For example:

- The facilities to subtract values of one CT image from those of the identical section through the body, imaged after the administration of a radiological contrast agent;
- Construction of sagittal, coronal and oblique sections from the data originally collected during the exposure of transverse scans through the same part of the body;
- Image enlargement;
- Edge enhancement.

### *Storage*

Storage may refer to currently collected data for immediate use in image construction, or to its retention for short-term, medium-term or archival duration. Either raw or processed and manipulated data can be stored. On completion of a CT examination and the patient's departure, permanent, long-term storage is provided on magnetic or optical discs.

### *Hard copies*

The image resulting from a CT scan may be documented by means of a hard copy – a photograph of the CT image on film or paper. The camera which produces such photographs typically operates in conjunction with a multiformat system, permitting several exposures to be made upon one subdivided sheet of film. Photographs may be filed and used as documentation of a patient's condition, but they cannot provide a record of an entire CT scan. Recall of all picture information is possible only from the memory stores associated with the computer. Retrieval from a disc can enable every facility for image manipulation to be repeated, provided that all the necessary data have been stored.

## 14.8 Image quality

Conventional radiographic images are judged according to their coverage of the required anatomical area, freedom from artefacts and two principal photographic criteria:

(1) Freedom from unsharpness – that is, demonstration of detail within the structure of the object;
(2) Contrast – that is, demonstration of the differences between various anatomical structures, particularly when they have different compositions and are situated adjacent to each other.

There are corresponding criteria by which CT images are assessed:

(1) Spatial resolution – that is, the ability to see small objects, separately defined.
(2) Sensitivity to tissue change – that is, ability to discriminate between adjacent structures on account of their density difference.

### *Spatial resolution*

This is determined by:

(1) The width of the detector apertures (normally 1.5–2 mm): the smaller this is, the greater the resolution.
(2) The matrix: the finer the matrix – that is, the larger the number of pixels – the greater the resolution.
(3) The slice thickness: thinner slices discriminate more clearly between fine structures, by giving more accurate CT numbers and reducing artefacts.
(4) The geometry of the system: focal spot size, tube–object and object–detector distances have effects as in conventional radiography.
(5) The computer program used for the reconstruction.
(6) The scanning speed: this affects reduction or elimination of motional

blur; and, because it influences the period of time during which photons may reach a detector it also affects the occurrence of quantum mottle.

## *Sensitivity to tissue change*

This is determined by:

(1) The X-ray beam quality – dependent on tube kilovoltage and filtration.
(2) Inherent quantum noise.
(3) Introduced electronic noise.
(4) The computer program used for the reconstruction.

### Resolution versus sensitivity

Spatial resolution and sensitivity to tissue change are complex subjects in CT. It may be that attempts to increase one can only be achieved at the expense of reducing the other.

To illustrate this potential conflict: in CT imaging, as in other radiographic imaging, the most challenging problem is posed by a small lesion presenting low contrast with its surroundings. In the demonstration of such a lesion, a system offering high spatial resolution may have difficulty due to a high level of quantum noise. Its ability to discriminate between different tissues may be limited by this noise (random behaviour of photons) so much that a small change in beam attenuation is undetectable because it produces a signal variation which is smaller than the noise. The signal-to-noise ratio can be improved by increasing the size of the aperture through which the X-ray beam is reaching a detector. The width of this aperture, however, fundamentally determines the resolution of a CT system. Thus one image quality factor conflicts with the other.

## *Radiation dose*

Any X-ray examination entails the administration of a radiation dose to a patient. Patient dose may be regarded as the total quantity of X-rays delivered to a patient. This will be minimized if the equipment and imaging system used possess high dose efficiency. This situation is obtained when all the X-rays which pass through a patient are converted to a usable signal.

The following features of CT scanners can account for photons emerging from the patient becoming *lost*, with consequently poor dose efficiency:

(1) If detectors are widely spaced, some photons will pass into the spaces between them.
(2) Inaccurate (insufficient) beam collimation may result in the projection of X-rays outside the area of the detector array.
(3) Information may be lost because the detectors themselves are ineffi-

cient. (Detector efficiency is a combination of photon collection and photon conversion to electrical current.)

To summarize: dose efficiency is the product of detector aperture, beam width and the photon conversion factor.

Dose efficiency is always an important parameter of performance in CT. During paediatric examinations, for example, it might be the most important consideration.

### Image quality versus radiation dose

In CT there is an intimate connection between radiation dose, spatial resolution and the accuracy with which absorption differences are detected and displayed. Images of high detail, with little noise, can be obtained only by increasing the amount of radiation. Thus, patient dose and image quality are factors to be balanced when equipment performance is to be assessed.

A high detail image is obtained by the use of a fine matrix; that is, through a proportional number of irradiations of many small anatomical voxels. Thus, there is a link between resolution and radiation dose: an image of high resolution is obtained by submitting the patient to a relatively high radiation dose.

Lack of clarity in a CT image originating from photon variations can be remedied if a larger number of photons is used. This means increasing the radiation dose and the number of X-rays crossing a voxel at different angles – that is, assuming optimum performance from the detectors. In this case, the equipment's sensitivity to tissue change has been increased at the cost of a higher dosage.

## 14.9 Use of CT equipment: the operator's judgement

There is a variety of CT equipment on the market. Ideally, CT equipment should allow the operator to balance the inter-related matters of resolution, sensitivity to tissue change and radiation dose against one another, in consideration of the needs of a particular clinical situation.

The potential conflict between factors influencing image quality have already been discussed. Skilled CT operators are aware of these and set imaging parameters in any given situation, in order to achieve optimum diagnostic information with minimum radiation hazards. Of course, this is of high importance in any situation involving exposure to ionizing radiations, but it may be especially so in relation to CT. The information which its images are capable of revealing can seduce a clinician, who does not appreciate the radiation hazards, into overusing it, even when equally effective and less harmful alternatives are available.

Questions which may be asked include:

- Is the probable lesion within an area of low contrast?
- Is high resolution really required?
- What radiation dose is justified?

Unfortunately, there is no mutual compatibility between all of these. Students will observe that skilled radiographers adjust the available resources, according to circumstances. For example:

(1) When examining an abdominal organ, an essential requirement may be the detectability of low contrasts.
(2) For skeletal examinations of the base of the skull, a thin section capability is needed.
(3) In dynamic scanning, the use of short scan times will be critically important.

## 14.10 Follow-up practical

Gain experience in studying at least two different CT units. Observe techniques and evaluate the equipment and its setting (the room or *suite*).

In evaluating CT equipment, absolute judgements should be avoided: the labels *good* and *bad* are unfortunate and potentially misleading. Equipment is purchased for particular reasons, and all need to be taken into account.

Points to look for are, obviously, the technical capabilities resulting from design features of the two units: gantry and table, X-ray facilities and computer – both hardware and software: for example, ability to perform dynamic scans, to image blood flow; to reconstruct coronal and sagittal sections from data collected during a sequence of transverse scans. There is the *user friendliness* of the controls, the units' reliability (how often are engineers called in for repairs?) and the ease with which the units can deal with a high workload. There is also the matter of purchase costs – huge sums, no doubt, which at the time had to be measured against other potential claims. Lastly, has age something to do with differences: what innovations were introduced during the interval between installation of the two units, and what will be the capabilities of eventual replacement equipment?

# Chapter 15
# Radionuclide Imaging

## 15.1 Introduction

Students who are familiar only with diagnostic radiography will need to adjust to the main principle of radionuclide imaging. The imaging radiation has its source within the patient's body; rays are emitted from (rather than transmitted through) the anatomical areas which are being studied. There is no equivalent to a radiographic projection. Instead, radiation emitted from within the body is detected externally in such a way that its origins – the anatomical site – can be clearly identified, to form an image. Images are formed by the radiation emitted from the body's surface nearest to the detector: thus an anterior (detected) image will differ from a posterior image.

Radionuclide imaging equipment provides a very sophisticated detecting and localizing system for radioactivity within the body. Before considering this equipment, it will be useful to look briefly at radioactivity and radionuclides.

## 15.2  Types of radioactivity

Radioactivity causes a radionuclide to transform into either another radionuclide or a stable nuclide. There are three types of radioactivity. Two are particulate in nature: subatomic alpha and beta particles are emitted. These cannot penetrate very far and would not reach a detector outside the body. Their only effect would be to give a radiation dose to the patient, for no diagnostic purpose.

The third type of radioactive decay results in the emission of **gamma radiation**. This is the emission employed to form images. At the same photon energies, gamma rays are identical to X-rays and thus possess equivalent penetrating powers.

The human body is composed of atoms which, for the most part, do not have radioactive isotopes suitable for imaging: their emissions, energies or half lives are inappropriate. It is therefore necessary for a radioactive material to be introduced temporarily into the body, to enable imaging to be carried out.

## 15.3 Choice of radionuclide

The radiation energy emitted from the patient must be sufficient for the rays to pass easily out of the body, but not so high that the imaging equipment would have difficulty in detecting (absorbing) it. Each radionuclide emits its own specific photon energy, i.e. the radiation is monoenergetic (homogeneous). The choice of radionuclide reflects a compromise between dose to the patient and ease of detection. In practice, this means that a radionuclide is chosen which emits photons with an energy value in the range 100–200 keV.

The radionuclide is introduced by being combined with a substance which will, in some appropriate way, be used by the body. The substance is described as having a radioactive **label** attached to it or, more simply, as having been labelled. Labelled substances which carry radioactivity are termed radiopharmaceuticals. After the introduction of a radiopharmaceutical into the body (usually by intravenous injection) its transport, uptake and distribution can be studied. The point may be made here, that whereas other modalities provide diagnostic information based on anatomy, radionuclide imaging reveals the physiology of the body or the selected organ. Its clinical importance lies in the fact that physiological changes may be apparent long before any structural changes become large enough to visualize.

Radiopharmaceuticals differ from other drugs, in that they:

(1) All contain a radionuclide;
(2) Are not administered in order to produce a pharmacological effect;
(3) Are given in *tracer* amounts, i.e. as a low percentage within a largely unlabelled volume, to reveal the movement and action of the whole.

The technique of using a tracer may be explained by the following analogy. If a check is to be made on the rate at which bricks are being used during the building of a house, it could be arranged for every hundredth brick to be painted blue. The task of counting the number of hundreds of bricks would then become simply a matter of counting the blue bricks. These blue bricks would still be bricks, i.e. they wouldn't weaken the house and the carefully chosen paint would disappear, after a while.

It must be pointed out that, although the radioactive tracer will decay and disappear, it will be the cause of a radiation dose to the patient. The magnitude of this dose is subject to radiation protection legislation controls.

## 15.4 Radiation dosimetry

If the body were to retain the radionuclide/radiopharmaceutical, the total dose would depend on its half life. A radionuclide with a short half life would be used, in order to minimize the dose to the patient. If, on the other hand, the radionuclide were to be rapidly excreted, a long half life would not present as much of a radiation hazard. There has to be a balance against the time needed to acquire the images. Generally, a higher dose of a short lived radionuclide is given, which produces a relatively high count rate (intensity) and relatively short acquisition (imaging) time.

Ideally, a radionuclide is required which will:

(1) Remain in the body for no longer than is necessary for completing the imaging process;
(2) Produce a high count rate while it is in the body;
(3) Be readily available;
(4) Not be too expensive.

Technetium 99m meets all these requirements. It is readily labelled onto several compounds, to produce radiopharmaceuticals for imaging most parts of the body and it can also be used without a carrier for some studies.

## 15.5 Technetium 99m

Technetium 99m is the daughter product of molybdenum (mass number 99) which has a half life of 67 hours. This means that a weekly supply of molybdenum 99 can be used in appropriate laboratory conditions to provide a daily supply of a sterile, radioactive solution of Technetium 99m.

The nuclear disintegration of a radionuclide gives rise to another nuclide with a different atomic number. Usually, any energy difference is lost simultaneously with the emitted subatomic particles. The symbol 'm' denotes a metastable nuclide. Metastable nuclides break up first and lose the energy at a later time. Technetium 99m has already undergone a nuclear transformation and only requires to shed its excess energy in the form of a gamma ray photon of 140 keV, for it to become stable (for practical purposes). It does this later. Thus it is a pure gamma emitter and, although all ionizing radiation has the potential to cause biological damage, it may be described as having good radiation dosimetry properties.

## 15.6 Equipment

The commonest item of equipment used in radionuclide imaging is a gamma camera. To understand its construction and operation, it is helpful, first, to look at one of its essential components.

*A scintillation crystal detector*

A single detector comprises a scintillation crystal which emits light flashes when it absorbs gamma ray photons, and a photomultiplier tube which converts light energy into a measurable electrical signal, proportional to the absorbed gamma ray energy. The crystal and photomultiplier tube are sealed into a lightproof aluminium housing which is lead lined, except at its input (crystal) end. Gamma radiation passes through the aluminium to strike the crystal, where some of its energy is absorbed. This causes emission of light. Behind the crystal and optically coupled to it, the photomultiplier tube releases electrons in proportion to the brightness of the scintillation. It is therefore energy sensitive.

The electron release is amplified by a series of electrodes, termed dynodes, at increasing positive potential. In succession, these attract and increase the electrons until a useful electrical pulse output is obtained. The greater the gamma ray energy absorbed, the brighter the scintillation and the larger the output signal from the photomultiplier tube. The maximum signal results when all the energy of the incoming photon is completely absorbed in one event, as opposed to a series of interactions. These devices are capable of very fast count rates with minimal loss.

The output from the photomultiplier tube is electronically analysed and usually displayed in one of two forms: as a readout of count rate (counts per second) or as a pulse height spectrum. A pulse height spectrum is produced when the brightness of each scintillation and its associated electrical pulse is measured by a pulse height (or multi-channel) analyser. This presents the information graphically, showing the peak emission of the source. If properly calibrated, it can be used to identify radionuclides by their specific photon energies.

If a detector has a lead collimator placed in front of it, the field of view, i.e. the area from which emitted radiation is being measured, is restricted. The device thus becomes more direction dependent. If it is placed close to the patient, it will only detect radiation emitted from a collimator sized area of the patient. With such a small field, the compilation of an image, showing the emissions from a part of the body (chest, abdomen, brain) is only possible by movement of the detector from point to point, i.e. by a scanning technique. The gamma camera is a device which achieves this same image instantly and can show changes occurring within it, in real time.

## 15.7 The gamma camera

The gamma camera comprises a large scintillation crystal which can receive radiation from a wide field via a multi-hole collimator, and to which (behind) are linked up to 60 or more photomultiplier tubes. This whole

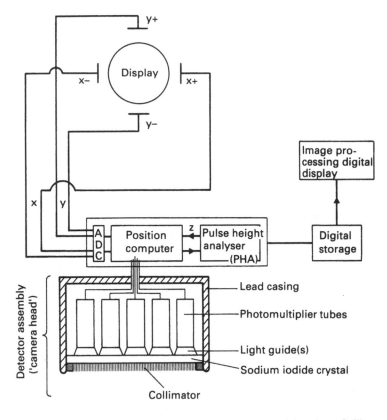

**Fig. 15.1** Schematic diagram of gamma camera and summary of functions. Collimator: allows radiation approaching its face at 90° (along the parallel axes of the holes) to pass through. Sodium iodide crystal: scintillates when exposed to radiation, with a brightness proportional to the radiation intensity. (The crystal is protected against light at the front.) Light guides: reduce light losses which would occur due to internal reflections, if there were gaps between the crystal and the photomultiplier tubes. Photomultiplier tubes: produce electric signals which are greatly amplified in proportion to the scintillation brightness. Position computer: uses all the simultaneous signals from a group of photomultiplier tubes to calculate where they are coming from, on the crystal face. These are added together to calculate the brightness of the scintillation. Pulse height analyser: can discriminate between signals which are of correct strength to form an image, and others which are either too weak (scatter) or too strong (due to two flashes occurring simultaneously). Operates within a preset tolerance, plus or minus the expected range. Its action, combined with the collimator, ensure accurate mapping of the radiation distribution within the patient. Analogue to digital converter (ADC): Digitizes the position co-ordinates and either displays them on a matrix or stores them for manipulation. Display: enables the position of the patient to be checked and monitored during acquisition.

detector assembly is lead shielded: radiation is allowed to enter only via the collimator. The area from which image-forming radiation is received may be circular or rectangular. A large camera will typically cover an area the size of a large X-ray film (35 cm × 43 cm) via a parallel hole collimator.

Due to attenuation within the crystal and the effect of the inverse square law, the strength of the pulses emitted from the photomultiplier tubes will vary. For practical purposes, however, they will respond simultaneously. A summation circuit and a position computer total the combined pulses, to arrive at values and positions for all the original scintillations.

A parallel hole collimator is constructed of lead foil or is a fine casting, in a honeycomb pattern. The walls (septa) marking out the pattern, have equal thickness, to allow even, maximum transmission of radiation through the open channels. The effect of the collimator, in selectively allowing radiation to reach the crystal, is similar to the action of a secondary radiation grid allowing transmission of primary X-rays, but blocking angled scatter. The thickness of the septa affects sensitivity and ability to cope with high energy. The depth of the holes affects spatial resolution. These two factors conflict, to some extent, necessitating a practical compromise. As in diagnostic radiography, gains in resolution are achieved at the expense of speed, and vice versa. There is an added dimension, however: time. The emission of radioactivity can be measured as it changes with time. The user of the camera must decide, in the circumstances, whether spatial or temporal resolution is more useful for securing a reliable diagnosis.

Radiation leaving the organ or area being investigated may interact with intervening body tissues, having its energy reduced by the Compton scattering process in proportion to the angle of direction change. The pulse height analyser is used to discriminate: it only allows pulses resulting from specified energies to be recorded. It can thus perform electronic removal of the scatter which travels along the axes of the collimator openings.

## Camera gantry

The gamma camera head is basically a lead box filled with delicate electronic detection equipment. It is extremely heavy (approximately 50 kg), requiring a strong support gantry but also needing to allow easy and accurate positioning, close to the patient's body. Collimators can be exchanged, to suit different imaging requirements and photon energies. This manoeuvre is easier and safer if a special trolley is available.

Sectional imaging techniques are increasingly entering radionuclide imaging. They require additional electronic facilities, but also the provision for the gamma camera head to be able to move around patients as they lie on the couch. For this, the gantry obviously needs to be more complex in its construction: the gamma camera head is motor driven and safety interlocks are built in with a *fail safe* provision, to prevent accidents.

## Couch

The patient support couch has a cantilever construction (rather than a

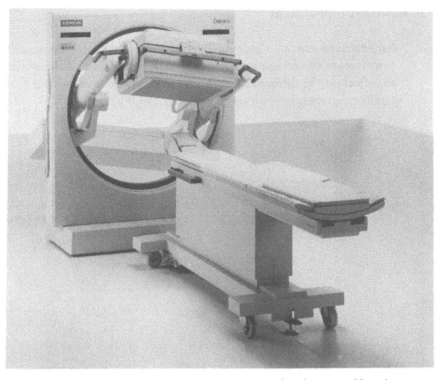

**Fig. 15.2** A modern, rectangular gamma camera, mounted on its gantry. Note the counterbalance to its weight. (*By courtesy of Siemens plc.*)

conventional supporting base or legs) to allow space underneath for the gamma camera head to record posterior emissions from a supine patient. The couch top is made of perspex and is commonly of the *floating* type. Some couches also have an adjustable height.

### Computer facilities

Radionuclide images are digitized and stored in computer memory. The major advantage of digitization is the ability actually to quantify the distribution of radioactivity and allow measurements to be made. An important facility is made possible with electrocardiograph or multiple gating: moving images can be produced of the beating heart, showing either the blood being pumped through the chambers or perfusion of cardiac muscle, depending on which radiopharmaceutical is employed. Multiple gating is a technique in which a time interval, such as a heart beat cycle, is subdivided into several equal time units. Radioactive disintegrations occurring during each time subdivision are recorded.

## 15.8 Follow-up practical

An extended visit to a radionuclide imaging department is essential if the principles of this imaging modality are to be appreciated. Students may care to reflect on the differences between radionuclide imaging and their more familiar experiences with diagnostic radiography.

# Chapter 16
# Equipment for Ultrasound Imaging

## 16.1 Introduction

Student radiographers now often become aware of ultrasound as early as during their first visit to a diagnostic imaging department (even though it may be referred to as an 'X-ray department'). Ultrasound's entry into the spectrum of imaging procedures, though fairly recent, has been comprehensive and very significant. It is probably best known for being the first choice imaging modality in the field of obstetrics, but it has a growing range of other applications. Both dynamic and static images can be produced and, as during a Doppler study, information can be displayed as a spectrum.

In some respects, ultrasound and X-rays may be considered complementary. Ultrasound tends to be more useful in areas where X-ray imaging is poor, but of little value in areas where X-ray imaging is excellent (see Table 16.1 for a comparison of the two techniques). For example, ultrasound is able to provide highly detailed images of abdominal organs such as the liver but is unsuitable for imaging bony structures or the lungs.

The technical differences between ultrasound and X-ray imaging are considerable, and there are many more differences than similarities. Both, however, use external sources of energy (high-frequency sound waves or X-rays), and depend upon interactions with tissue to produce images. Additionally – and significantly – both imaging modalities impose a requirement on radiographers to understand the equipment producing the relevant energy, the interactions which occur, and the imaging processes. These needs and the growing range of clinical applications, confirm that student radiographers must include ultrasound in their studies of *Equipment*.

## 16.2 Basic functions of ultrasound imaging equipment

Ultrasound is high frequency, inaudible sound. For medical imaging procedures, the frequencies most commonly used are in the range 3 MHz to 10 MHz. Being a mechanical or vibrational energy, unlike X-rays which, being an electromagnetic radiation, can cross a vacuum, ultrasound requires

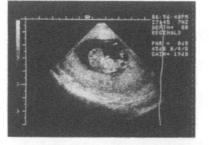

(a)

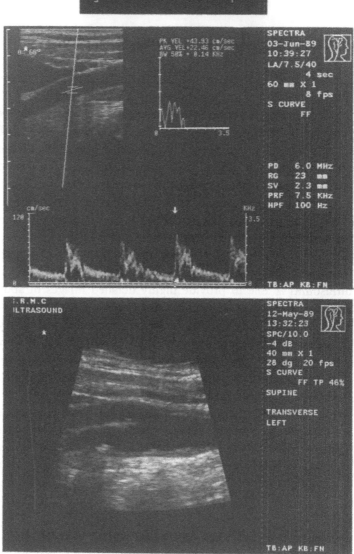

(b)

(c)

Fig. 16.1 (a) An ultrasound image of a fetus. Recorded during a dynamic (real time) examination, using a grey scale B-mode imaging system. (*Courtesy of Acuson Ltd.*) (b) A Doppler spectrum of the common carotid artery. Mixed mode display of the common carotid artery. Obtained by use of 7.5 MHz flat linear array probe with steerable Doppler cursor. (*Courtesy of Diasonics Sonotron.*) (c) Image of the common carotid artery, showing irregular thickening of anterior and posterior walls. (*Courtesy of Diasonics Sonotron.*)

**Table 16.1** Comparison of ultrasound and X-ray imaging.

| Ultrasound imaging | X-ray imaging |
| --- | --- |
| Uses a mechanical energy source which is non-ionizing | Uses an electromagnetic ionizing radiation |
| Depends on interaction processes within tissue | Depends on interaction processes within tissue |
| Produces images as a result of ultrasound energy being reflected and scattered within the body | Produces images as a result of X-rays being absorbed within the body |
| At the power levels used has not demonstrated any adverse bio-effects | Produces well documented biological effects in tissue |
| Demonstrates structure of soft tissues and organs well | Does not demonstrate soft tissues and organs well |
| Is able to discriminate between structures with only small density differences | Using conventional X-ray imaging, relatively large differences in density are required in order to discriminate between structures |
| Ultrasound requires a medium in which to propagate | X-rays propagate in a vacuum as well as in a medium |
| The speed of ultrasound varies according to the medium in which it is propagating and is a constant for any given medium | The speed at which X-rays propagate is unimportant in X-ray imaging |
| Ultrasound energy is attenuated exponentially | X-radiation intensity is, for practical purposes, attenuated exponentially |

a medium for its propagation. Production of an ultrasound image begins when ultrasound is transmitted into a medium by a transducer. Some of this ultrasound energy is returned to the transducer and then processed to form ultrasound images or other recognizable information displays.

The functions of ultrasound imaging equipment may therefore be summarized as:

(1) To initiate and control the production of ultrasound energy.
(2) To enable the ultrasound energy to be transmitted into a medium.
(3) To receive, manipulate, process and display, in the required form, the proportion of the ultrasound energy that is returned from the medium to the transducer.

### Pulse-echo imaging

Pulse-echo imaging requires a pulse of ultrasound to be generated by a transducer and propagated into tissue. Within tissue, the ultrasound pulse

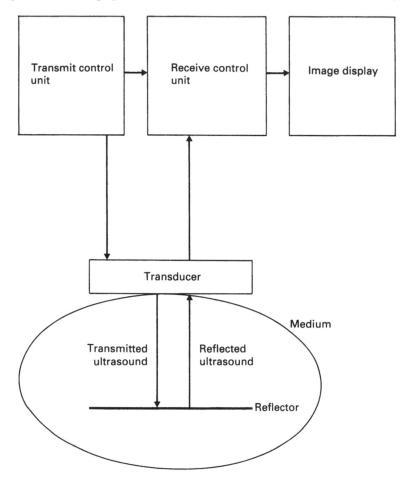

**Fig. 16.2** Block diagram to demonstrate the basic functions of ultrasound imaging equipment.

interacts with reflecting boundaries or targets which return some of the ultrasound energy to the transducer, where a signal is generated. The time period between generation of the ultrasound pulse and detection of its reflection is measured accurately. This enables the distance between transducer and reflector to be calculated and thus the depth within the tissue from which the reflection has been produced.

The strength of the signal generated at a transducer by a returning ultrasound beam will vary according to the beam's intensity. Signal magnitude thus provides information about the nature of the reflectors from which such signals arise: strong reflectors produce large (high amplitude) signals and weak reflectors produce small (low amplitude) ones.

Signals arising from tissue therefore contain both depth and amplitude information, particularly to specific reflection boundaries or targets within

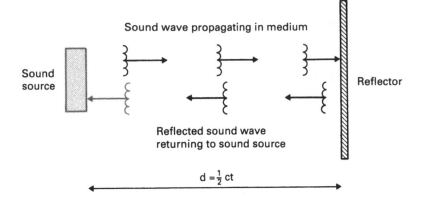

**Fig. 16.3** The principles of pulse-echo ultrasound imaging. d = distance between sound source and reflector; c = speed of sound in the medium; t = time taken for sound to travel from the source to the reflector and back again to the source.

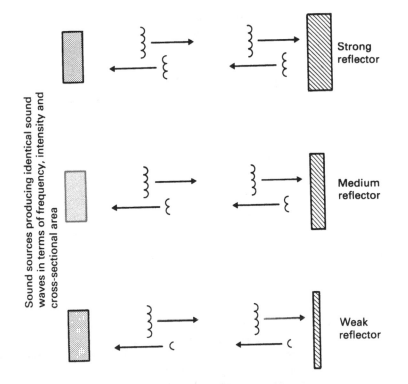

**Fig. 16.4** The nature of reflectors and signal strength. Note that as the reflector becomes weaker, the intensity of the reflected ultrasound beam decreases. Thus, signal magnitude (reflected intensity) provides information about the nature of the reflector from which a signal arises.

the tissue. The receive/control unit now manipulates these signals so that an image of the tissue may be produced and displayed in an analogue form.

## 16.3 The nature of ultrasound and its propagation in human tissue

The functions of ultrasound imaging equipment can only be appreciated fully if the nature of ultrasound waves and their propagation in human tissue are understood.

*Propagation of ultrasound in tissue*

Ultrasound waves result from the mechanical disturbance of a particulate medium. In diagnostic medical imaging, this medium is human tissue.

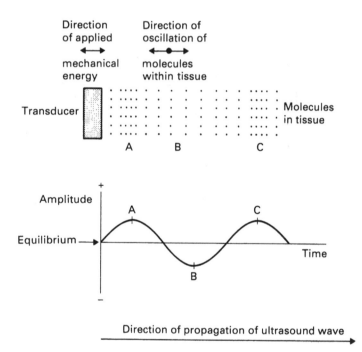

**Fig. 16.5** Continuous, sinusoidal, longitudinal ultrasound wave motion. Mechanical disturbance arising from a transducer makes molecules of the tissue, with which it is in contact, oscillate about their normal positions. A and C correspond to regions in which molecules are pushed *close together*, due to the relative oscillations of adjacent individual molecules, i.e. areas of *compression* or excess positive pressure within the tissue. B corresponds to a region in which the molecules are *pulled furthest apart*, i.e. an area of *rarefaction* or excess negative pressure. The repetition of this process sets up a sinusoidally varying, longitudinal wave motion by which ultrasound energy is transmitted through the tissue.

Mechanical disturbance arising from a **transducer** causes particles (i.e. molecules) within the human tissue with which it is in contact to vibrate or oscillate about their normal positions. As the molecules immediately adjacent to the source of the mechanical disturbance oscillate, they interact with neighbouring molecules. In turn, these too begin to oscillate. This process is repeated and a sinusoidally varying, longitudinal wave motion is generated within the tissue, so transmitting ultrasound energy through the tissue. The direction of ultrasound wave propagation and energy flow is along the same axis as the direction of motion of the molecules. Ultrasound energy will propagate continuously in this manner for as long as a mechanical disturbance is applied to the tissue.

## Ultrasound wave parameters

The sinusoidal shape of a continuous ultrasound wave enables its parameters to be described easily. These are:

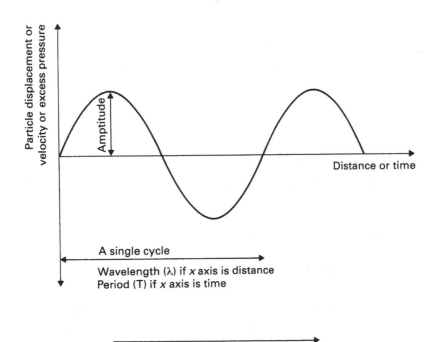

**Fig. 16.6** Continuous ultrasound waveform parameters. On this graph, the vertical (*y*) axis may represent particle displacement, particle velocity or particle excess pressure; and the horizontal (*x*) axis may represent distance or time. Note that while pressure and displacement are in phase, velocity is 90° out of phase with both. (Frequency (*f*) is the number of complete cycles passing a given point in 1 second – cycles per second (cps) or hertz (Hz).)

- **Wavelength** or period;
- **Amplitude**, which may represent particle displacement, particle velocity or particle excess pressure;
- **Frequency**.

There are a number of diagnostic medical ultrasound units, particularly for investigating blood flow and fetal heart function, which use continuously propagating ultrasound waves as described above. These are known as **continuous wave** (CW) ultrasound machines.

In pulse-echo ultrasound imaging equipment, however, the ultrasound beam is not propagated continuously but is *pulsed in very short bursts.* Typically, a pulse-echo system will generate ultrasound pulses of 1 μs at a repetition rate of 1000 pulses per second.

### *Speed of ultrasound*

It has been established that ultrasound energy propagates or travels through tissue as a result of the relative motion of adjacent molecules within tissue, when under the influence of an applied source of mechanical energy. The speed with which ultrasound energy propagates through any medium is dependent upon inherent properties of the medium. *Speed* of propagation is thus a *constant for any given medium.* The properties which determine it are the density and the elasticity of the material. These are related by the formula:

$$c = \left(\frac{E}{\rho}\right)^{½}$$

where

$c$ = speed of ultrasound in a given medium
$E$ = elastic modulus or stiffness of the medium
$\rho$ = density of the medium

Human tissue is heterogeneous in its composition, i.e. it is made up of a range of different tissues, for example: blood, water, fat, muscle, bone. Discrete organs within the body contain differing combinations of these tissues, hence the speed of ultrasound in the human body varies according to the type of tissue or the organ or structure in which it is propagating. The speed of ultrasound through the various soft tissues of the human body does not vary greatly, however, so it is possible to derive a useful average value for human soft tissue.

## 16.4 Interactions of ultrasound energy and tissue

When ultrasound energy is propagated in human tissue, a number of interactions occur which together enable ultrasound images to be produced.

**Table 16.2** Speed of sound in various media.

| Medium | Speed in metres per second |
|---|---|
| Soft tissue (average) | 1540 |
| Blood | 1570 |
| Fat | 1460 |
| Muscle | 1580 |
| Bone | 3500 |
| Liver | 1570 |
| Kidney | 1560 |
| Lung | 650 |
| Water (20° C) | 1480 |
| Air | 330 |

The important interactions are **specular reflection** and **scatter** or **non-specular reflection**.

In general terms, it may be said that *specular reflection* enables *boundaries* (organ capsules, vessel walls, etc.) to be imaged, while *scatter* interactions take place within the *substance* of organs and structures, so enabling parenchymal tissue to be imaged.

Other interactions – notably **refraction** and **absorption**, as well as the process of **attenuation** – affect the production of ultrasound images. These need to be taken into consideration during the design and use of ultrasound imaging equipment.

### Acoustic impedance

The term **acoustic impedance** is an important factor in understanding ultrasound interactions and the design of equipment. The acoustic impedance of a medium may be said to represent the difficulty with which ultrasound energy is able to travel through that medium. Like speed of sound, acoustic impedance is (a) a constant for any given medium, and (b) dependent on the density and elasticity of the medium. It is determined fundamentally by the relationship:

$$Z = \frac{P_p}{P_v}$$

where

$Z$ = acoustic impedance
$P_p$ = particle (excess) pressure
$P_v$ = particle velocity

As the excess pressure experienced by particles in a medium, and their velocities are difficult quantities to measure, it is more convenient to express acoustic impedance as:

$$Z = \rho c$$

where

$Z$ = acoustic impedance
$\rho$ = density of the medium
$c$ = speed of ultrasound within the medium

## Specular reflection

Specular reflection occurs when the ultrasound beam is incident on a *smooth* interface, which is relatively large compared to the wavelength of the beam, lying between two media of differing acoustic impedances. At such an interface, only part of the incident ultrasound is transmitted; part is reflected from the interface, back through the first medium, and so does not pass into the second medium.

The angle at which ultrasound is reflected from the smooth interface is always equal to its angle of incidence.

In cases of smooth interface reflection, the *difference between the acoustic impedances* of the two media determines the relative intensities of the reflected and the transmitted ultrasound.

For an ultrasound beam meeting an interface at right angles, this relationship is expressed by the formulae:

$$R = \frac{I_r}{I_i} = \left(\frac{Z_2 - Z_1}{Z_1 + Z_2}\right)^2$$

and

$$T = \frac{I_t}{I_i} = \frac{4Z_1 \cdot Z_2}{(Z_1 + Z_2)^2}$$

where

$R$ = reflection intensity coefficient
$T$ = transmission intensity coefficient
$I_r$ = reflected ultrasound intensity
$I_t$ = transmitted ultrasound intensity
$Z_1$ = acoustic impedance of first medium
$Z_2$ = acoustic impedance of second medium

For an ultrasound beam that is incident non-normally, the intensities of the reflected and transmitted ultrasound beams are determined not only by

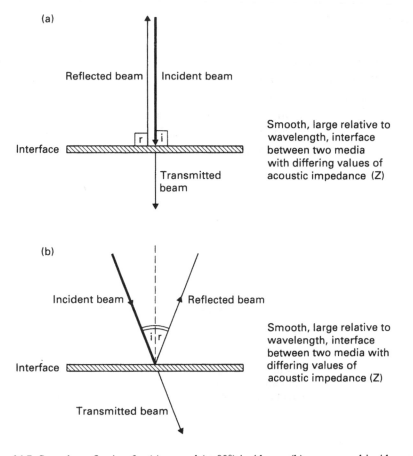

**Fig. 16.7** Specular reflection for (a) normal (at 90°) incidence; (b) non-normal incidence. The interface marks the boundary between two media of differing acoustic impedances (*Z*); it is smooth and large in relation to the ultrasound's wavelength. Note that, in both cases, the angle (*r*) through which ultrasound is reflected from a smooth interface is equal to the angle (*i*) of incidence.

the acoustic impedances of the media at the interface, but also by the angle of incidence.

The proportion of ultrasound energy reflected depends on the difference between the values of acoustic impedance (*Z*) in the two media forming the interface, such that the greater the difference, the greater will be the proportion of ultrasound energy reflected. For example, almost total reflection will occur from an interface between air and human tissue because their acoustic impedance values are markedly different, while almost total transmission occurs between kidney and perinephric fat, where their values differ only slightly.

Whenever specular reflection occurs, some loss of energy from the propagating ultrasound beam will occur.

## Scatter

Scatter is the other important interaction. It occurs when ultrasound is incident on a *rough* surface or on particles that are small in comparison with the wavelength of the incident ultrasound; for example, within soft tissues: fetal brain tissue, liver, etc.

When ultrasound strikes a small tissue particle, most of the incident ultrasound energy will pass onwards unchanged. A small proportion, however, interacts with the particle and is scattered in all directions. Thus,

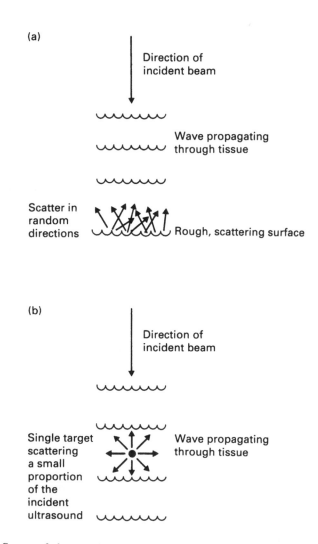

**Fig. 16.8** Scatter of ultrasound (a) from a rough surface; (b) from a single particle. When ultrasound strikes a rough surface (a) it is scattered in random directions. On striking a single, small tissue particle (b) most of it passes onwards unchanged with only a small proportion scattered – although this travels in all directions, including back to the source.

some of the ultrasound energy is scattered backwards in the direction of the ultrasound source.

Scatter interactions cause energy to be lost from the propagating ultrasound beam. As the frequency of the ultrasound beam increases, so too does the energy lost from the propagating beam. This is an important factor to consider when selecting an ultrasound frequency during scanning.

## Other interactions

### Refraction
Refraction also occurs at the boundary between two media. In contrast to specular reflection, however, it depends on a *change in the speed of sound* between the two media rather than a change in the values of acoustic impedance.

When the speed of sound changes at a boundary and the angle of incidence of the ultrasound beam is non-normal, the transmitted ultrasound

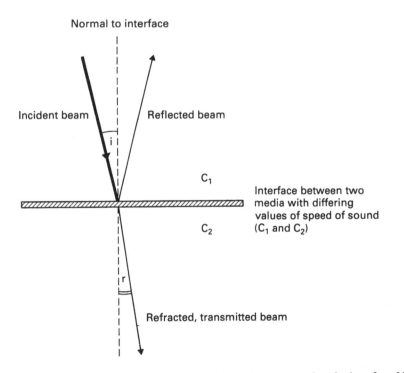

**Fig. 16.9** Principles of refraction. The incident beam is non-normal to the interface. Note that refraction occurs at a boundary where there is a difference between the *speed of sound* in the two media. An instance is shown where the speed in the first medium ($c_1$) is greater than in the second ($c_2$); deviation is towards the normal. In cases where the speed is less in the first medium than in the second, deviation is away from the normal.

beam deviates from its original path. The degree of deviation is determined by Snell's Law:

$$\frac{\sin i}{\sin r} = \frac{C_1}{C_2}$$

where

$\sin i$ = sine of the angle of incidence
$\sin r$ = sine of the angle of refraction
$C_1$ = speed of sound in the first medium
$C_2$ = speed of sound in the second medium

The *direction* of deviation of the transmitted beam depends on whether the ultrasound is passing from a medium in which the speed of sound is fast in relation to the second medium or vice versa. If the speed of sound in the first medium is fast relative to the speed of sound in the second medium, the deviation will be towards the normal. Deviation will be away from the normal if the speed of sound in the first medium is slow compared to in the second medium.

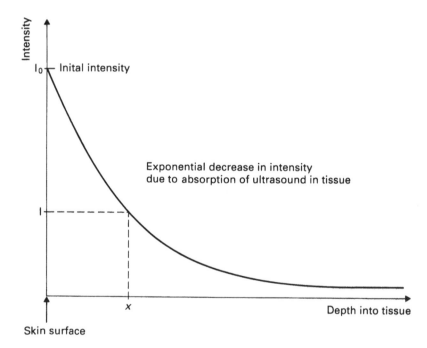

**Fig. 16.10** Exponential absorption of ultrasound. Absorption occurs exponentially, being dependent on ultrasound frequency: as frequency increases so does the loss of energy.

$$I = I_0 e^{-\mu_a x}$$

where $I$ = intensity at depth $x$ in the tissue; $I_0$ = intensity at the skin surface (zero depth); $\mu_a$ = absorption coefficient; $x$ = depth in tissue at which $I$ is measured.

## Absorption

Absorption is a complex process whereby some of the mechanical energy of the ultrasound beam is converted into heat energy, so reducing the intensity of the propagating beam. In soft tissue imaging, the process of absorption is the greatest cause of loss of energy from the propagating ultrasound beam.

Absorption occurs exponentially. It is also dependent on the frequency of the propagating ultrasound beam such that, for a specific medium, as frequency increases so does the loss of energy.

## Attenuation

A number of processes which reduce the intensity of an ultrasound beam passing through a medium have been described. The summative effect of

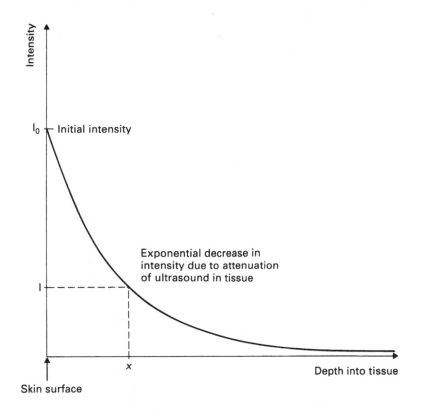

**Fig. 16.11** Ultrasound attenuation in tissue. Attenuation is the decrease in amplitude and intensity experienced by an ultrasound wave as it travels through tissue. Like absorption, it occurs exponentially and is frequency dependent. Note that the rate of decrease in intensity is greater than in Fig. 16.10.

$$I = I_0 e^{-\mu x}$$

where $I$ = intensity at depth $x$ in the tissue; $I_0$ = intensity at the skin surface; $\mu$ = attenuation coefficient; $x$ = depth in the tissue at which $I$ is measured.

these (as well as any other mechanisms which reduce beam intensity) is known as **attenuation**. Attenuation may be defined as the decrease in amplitude and intensity experienced by an ultrasound wave as it propagates in tissue. Like absorption, attenuation occurs exponentially and is frequency dependent.

## 16.5  Core modules of ultrasound equipment

Many different ultrasound imaging units are available, ranging widely in price and application, from simple A-Mode imaging to colour duplex imaging. Despite these considerable differences, all units rely upon similar sets of core modules. There are five major functional modules, each made up from a large number of discrete parts. Their number increases with the complexity of the equipment.

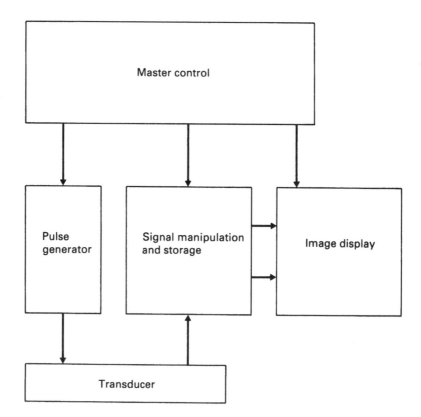

**Fig. 16.12** Block diagram of core modules in ultrasound imaging equipment.

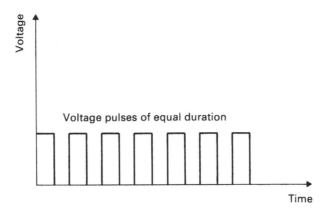

**Fig. 16.13** Low voltage, square wave form from the master control unit. The series of low voltage square wave pulses is generated at regular time intervals, so providing a highly accurate clock or timing device.

## Master control

The master control co-ordinates the functions of the whole ultrasound imaging unit. It generates a series of low voltage, square wave pulses at regular time intervals, so providing a highly accurate clock or timing device. Due to the nature of its function, the master control is also referred to as the **pulse repetition frequency generator**, as its voltage pulses are generated at a pre-determined frequency.

The leading edge of each voltage pulse simultaneously:

(1) Causes the pulse generator to trigger the transducer;
(2) Activates the signal manipulation and storage module (in particular the time–gain compensation unit); and
(3) Starts the image display equipment.

## Pulse generator

The pulse generator in its simplest form produces high voltage pulses which energize the transducer under the control of the master control module. Each voltage pulse causes the transducer to produce a single pulse of ultrasound.

## Transducer

An ultrasound transducer has two functions. It is a device which is able to change electrical signals into mechanical energy, so *generating* an ultrasound wave and setting up mechanical or vibrational disturbances of molecules in the medium immediately adjacent to it. Secondly, a transducer is able to

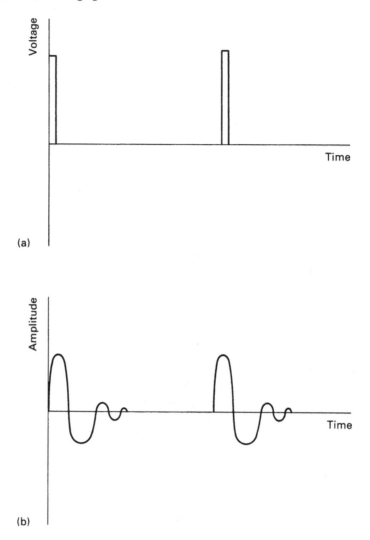

**Fig. 16.14** (a) Voltage pulses from the pulse generator to the transducer. (b) Resultant short pulses of ultrasound (1μs or less) emitted from the transducer.

*detect* ultrasound that has been reflected from the medium, and convert it into an electrical signal.

### Piezoelectricity

Ultrasound transducers function because they are piezoelectric materials. The properties of such materials are:

(1) They deform when an electric field is applied to them – the **inverse piezoelectric effect**; and
(2) Conversely, if they are subject to external pressure which causes them to deform, they will generate an electric potential across their surfaces – the **piezoelectric effect**.

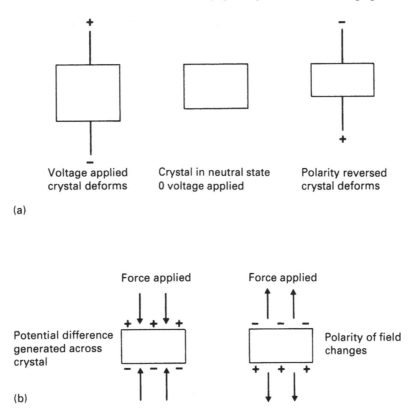

**Fig. 16.15** (a) The inverse piezoelectric effect. (b) The piezoelectric effect.

### Piezoelectricity and ultrasound transducers

Piezoelectric materials can occur naturally; quartz is an example. Transducers found in ultrasound imaging equipment, however, are normally made from artificially produced ceramics, specially treated to give them piezoelectric properties. The most common of these is **lead zirconate titanate** (usually referred to as **PZT**). Another material used as a transducer is polyvinylidine difluoride (PVDF).

In ultrasound imaging, the transducer is pulsed with a voltage from the pulse generator. As it deforms, under the effect of these pulses, the transducer causes a disturbance of molecules in the medium adjacent to it and thus propagates an ultrasound wave. Ultrasound is generated, therefore, in accordance with the inverse piezoelectric effect.

When ultrasound energy, reflected from tissues, returns to the transducer, it exerts pressure so that the transducer deforms. When this occurs, the transducer exhibits the piezoelectric effect: an electrical potential is generated across it.

Ultrasound transducers are fundamental to the construction and operation of ultrasound imaging equipment – so much so that, of the five essential modules, the transducer may be regarded as the most important. This point is often overlooked by staff who carelessly handle the probes housing the transducers, dropping them or leaving them covered in acoustic coupling gel.

### Signal manipulation and storage

This core module varies considerably from machine to machine, generally becoming more complex as the range of features offered on a machine

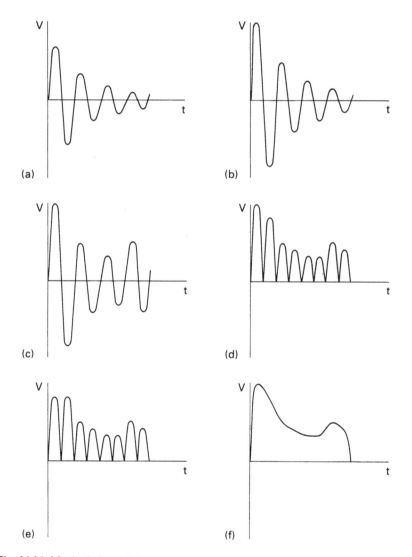

**Fig. 16.16** Manipulations of the voltage signal generated at the transducer. (a) Voltage signal generated by echo returning from tissue; (b) linear amplification; (c) differential amplification; (d) rectification; (e) high frequency filtering; (f) smooth envelope output from demodulator.

increases. Regardless of its complexity, however, this module performs some standard functions:

- Linear amplification of the voltage signals generated at the transducer by reflections (echoes) from tissue. A radio frequency (RF) amplifier is used for this purpose, as the signals generated are in the RF range.
- Amplitude limitation to protect the RF amplifier from very large transmitted ultrasound pulses.
- Differential amplification of the voltage signals generated at the transducer, according to the depth in tissue from which the echoes arise. This is necessary in order to counteract the effects of attenuation on both the propagating ultrasound beam and the returning echoes. Differential amplification is carried out by a **time–gain compensator (TGC)** applying a control voltage to the RF amplifier. The process is controlled by the master control: at the same time as it triggers the pulse generator, it also triggers the TGC. The TGC generates a control voltage (applied to the RF amplifier) that increases exponentially during the period in which the transducer is receiving echoes from tissue.
- Demodulation of the amplified voltage signal. First this signal is rectified. Then it is filtered to remove the highest frequency components. Filtering of very low frequency components may also take place. The signal output after demodulation is a smooth, envelope signal corresponding to the signal generated by echoes received at the transducer.
- Demodulator output signal digitization and storage. The signal may also be subject to a variety of manipulations either before digitization and storage or afterwards. In most modern ultrasound units, sophisticated computer technology now controls these functions. The image storage part of this module also provides facilities for image recording.

### Image display

Invariably, this is a television monitor which displays a visual image of the echo information from tissue. Most ultrasound units have monochrome (black and white) monitors which enable grey scale images to be displayed optimally. Increasingly, however, machines are providing facilities for colour imaging of blood flow and therefore require colour monitors.

## 16.6 Modes of ultrasound imaging

The various clinical applications of ultrasound depend on the mode in which it is used. While the fundamental principles of ultrasound beam production, propagation, reflection and reception are similar for all modes, the manipulations to which the received signals (echoes) are subject differ considerably, so producing very different images. The modes most commonly encountered are:

- **A-mode** (or amplitude-modulated mode).
- **B-mode** (or brightness-modulated mode). This is the most frequently

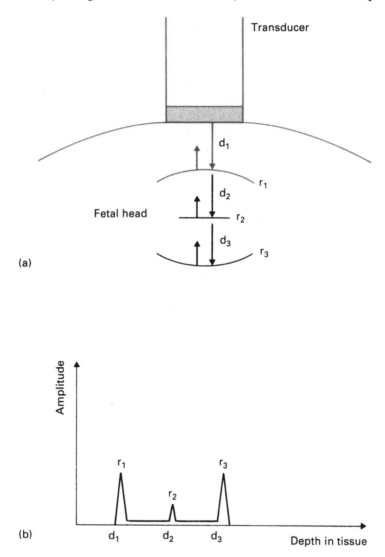

**Fig. 16.17** Principles of A-mode scanning. (a) Scan of a fetal head; $d_1$ = distance from skin surface to fetal skull ($r_1$); $d_2$ = distance from fetal skull to midline structure ($r_2$); $d_3$ = distance from midline structure to fetal skull ($r_3$). (b) Resultant image display. The image is a graph of echo amplitude plotted against arrival time at the transducer, displayed to represent the depth within the tissue from which the echoes arise. *Note:* A-mode scanning detects reflections from specular reflectors, i.e. large, smooth interfaces, marking a significant change in acoustic impedance.

used and versatile ultrasound imaging mode, forming the basis of all real time ultrasound imaging equipment and its applications.

- **M-mode** (or motion mode). An alternative and more accurate term (although it has fallen into disuse) is time–position, or TP mode.
- The **Doppler** effect.

## *Principles of A-mode scanning (see Fig. 16.17 opposite)*

In A-mode operation, the image is produced in the form of a graph: the amplitude of the echoes received at the transducer are displayed against their time of arrival at the transducer, such that the time base represents the depth in tissue from which the echoes arise.

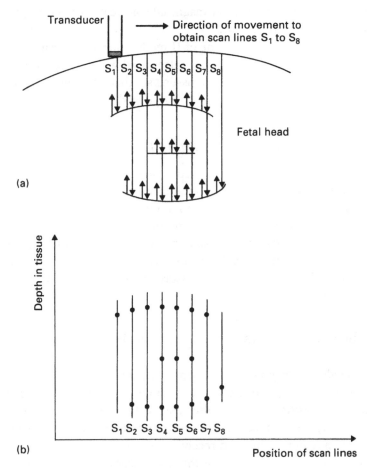

**Fig. 16.18** Principles of B-mode scanning. Images are built up from sequential lines of B-mode information, obtained as the ultrasound beam is systematically moved across the tissue. (a) B-scan of fetal head; (b) resultant image display. The echoes' amplitudes are represented by spots along each scan line, the degree of each spot's brightness corresponding to the magnitude of the received echo.

Applications of A-mode scanning are now quite limited. There is one important application, however: in measuring the axial length of the eye. This is performed in order to gauge the precise size of artificial lens implants, prior to lens implant surgery. Dedicated, highly automated units are used which both carry out the scanning and compute the size of implant directly, so minimizing the risks of error (particularly human).

### *Principles of B-mode scanning (see Fig. 16.18 on page 239)*

The widely-used B-mode is a development of A-mode. Initially, the amplitude trace is converted to a single bright spot positioned on the time base of the graph, with its brightness corresponding to the amplitude. Thus, the greater the amplitude or magnitude of the returned echo, the brighter is the spot on the time base.

This produces a single line of B-mode information from the tissue being examined. A mechanism is now introduced which systematically moves the ultrasound beam across the tissue, so that sequential lines of B-mode information are obtained and an image of the tissue is built up.

### *Principles of M-mode scanning (see Fig. 16.19 opposite)*

M-mode scanning is also derived from a simple A-scan line. This is again converted into a B-scan line, but information from this line is now collected over a period of time which may range from a few seconds to several minutes. Stationary targets from the tissue being scanned maintain a constant position along the scan line over time, while moving targets change their position over time. Thus, the image shows *stationary* targets as *straight* lines, while *moving* targets are displayed as *varying* lines.

## 16.7  Probes, transducers and ultrasound beam shapes

Transducers may be single or multi-element. They are mounted within a rugged housing and are the key components of ultrasound probes. The terms **transducer** and **probe** tend to be used interchangeably. Strictly, however, the transducer is the piezoelectric element responsible for producing ultrasound and receiving echoes from tissue, while the probe is the whole assembly in which the transducer element is housed.

The range of probes available currently is considerable and continues to grow. Probes now available include a wide range designed for conventional, **real time** scanning (e.g. abdominal and obstetric scanning); **intracavitary** scanning (e.g. transrectal, transvaginal and transurethral scanning); **intra-**

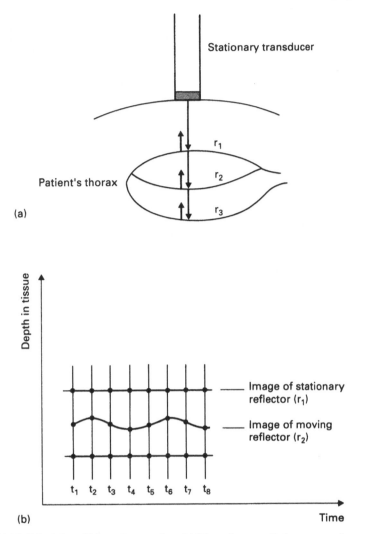

**Fig. 16.19** Principles of M-mode scanning. (a) M-mode scan of a heart; $r_1$ and $r_3$ are static reflectors; $r_2$ (heart valve) is a moving reflector that moves rhythmically towards and away from the transducer. (b) Resultant image display. The transducer remains in a fixed position but emits successive ultrasound pulses at fixed intervals. Each ultrasound pulse produces a scan line ($t_1$ to $t_8$) and enables the motion of the reflector to be imaged (stationary targets being shown as straight lines; moving targets as varying lines).

**operative** scanning (e.g. neurosurgical procedures); **endoscopic** scanning (e.g. trans-oesophageal scanning); and **intra-arterial** scanning.

### Construction of a single-element ultrasound probe

While not commonly found in modern ultrasound imaging equipment, single-element transducers provide a useful model for considering the basic

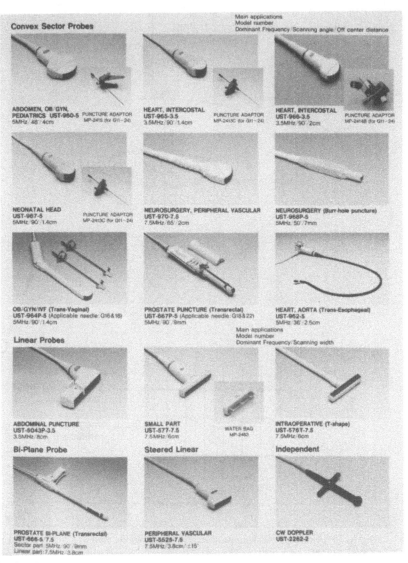

**Fig. 16.20** Ultrasound probes currently available. (*Courtesy of Aloka Co Ltd.*) Note that the range of probes continues to grow: for conventional real time, intracavitary, intraoperative, endoscopic and intra-arterial scanning.

design characteristics of all ultrasound transducers and ultrasound beam shapes.

### The transducer element
The disc of material forming the transducer element has been polarized permanently across its thickness to give it piezoelectric properties. It may be made flat or shaped and its diameter will also be determined, according to the ultrasound beam shape required and the application for which the probe

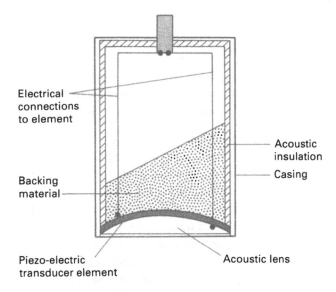

Electrical connections to element

Backing material

Piezo-electric transducer element

Acoustic insulation

Casing

Acoustic lens

**Fig. 16.21** Construction of a single-element transducer. The wedge–shaped rear surface of the backing material ensures that reflections from it are directed away from the transducer element, so that they cannot interfere with the ultrasound produced in response to the voltage pulse generator.

is to be used. Typical diameters range between 5 mm and 20 mm. The thickness of the element will determine the operating frequency of the transducer. Typical element thicknesses range from 0.2 mm to 2.0 mm. Silver electrodes are deposited on the front and rear surfaces, providing connection to the pulse generator so that the transducer element may be pulsed.

### Matching layer

A matching layer, which may be single or multiple, is positioned in front of the piezoelectric disc. Its purpose is to help overcome the acoustic mismatch between the piezoelectric disc and human tissue. PZT, the most common of the ceramics used as ultrasound transducers, has an acoustic impedance approximately 14 times greater than the acoustic impedance of human soft tissue. Such a large mismatch in acoustic impedance between materials forming a boundary will cause a large proportion of incident ultrasound to be reflected. If this were permitted to occur at the transducer/tissue interface, very little of the ultrasound produced would enter the tissue. Materials used for matching layers have acoustic impedance values that are the geometric mean of the values for the materials which, in use, lie on either side: the particular piezoelectric material and human tissue, as in the formula:

$$Z_m = (Z_e \cdot Z_t)^{1/2}$$

where

$Z_m$ = acoustic impedance of the matching layer material
$Z_e$ = acoustic impedance of the transducer element
$Z_t$ = acoustic impedance of human soft tissue

Materials used include epoxy resins, perspex and silicone rubber.

While matching layers assist in reducing the acoustic mismatch between the transducer element and human tissue, it is also necessary to *exclude air from the probe/tissue interface*; the difference in acoustic impedance between the matching layer and even a thin film of air between probe and tissue would result in most of the transmitted ultrasound being reflected before it entered the tissue. **Coupling materials**, typically water soluble gels with acoustic impedances of intermediate values between those of matching layer materials and human tissue, are used for this purpose.

A matching layer may be shaped to form an ultrasound beam focusing lens. Its thickness may also be controlled precisely to $\lambda/4$ to maximize the ultrasound energy transfer from the transducer element to the tissue.

### Backing layer

A backing layer is required for any transducer element which produces pulses of ultrasound. Its effect is to reduce the duration of the ultrasound pulses by *damping emissions from the rear surface* of the transducer element. This improves the spatial resolution properties of the ultrasound beam along its length (its axial resolution).

The materials used are epoxy resins loaded with metal powders, typically Araldite loaded with tungsten powder. The materials have two main features. Firstly, they have a similar acoustic impedance to the transducer element, so ensuring maximum transmission of ultrasound from the element into the backing layer. Secondly, being packed with small scattering targets (the metal powder) there is high absorption of ultrasound energy. Hence, the backing layer attenuates ultrasound very rapidly. In addition, the rear surface of the backing layer may be wedge shaped. This ensures that reflections from the surface are directed away from the transducer element and so are unable to interfere with the ultrasound produced by the applied voltage from the pulse generator.

### Casing

The probe's casing must be electrically and acoustically isolated from the transducer element. This arrangement maintains the element's acoustic efficiency (or sensitivity). A modern probe normally has a plastic casing with a built-in metallic screening layer.

The casing must be designed to allow for connection of the probe to the remainder of the unit, ease of use and cleaning, and be able to withstand the constant handling to which it will be exposed during use.

**Ultrasound beam characteristics from a single-element transducer**
The simplest transducer element is a flat circular disc of finite diameter and thickness. A more complex shape is required for pulsed ultrasound but, even so, the general features are similar.

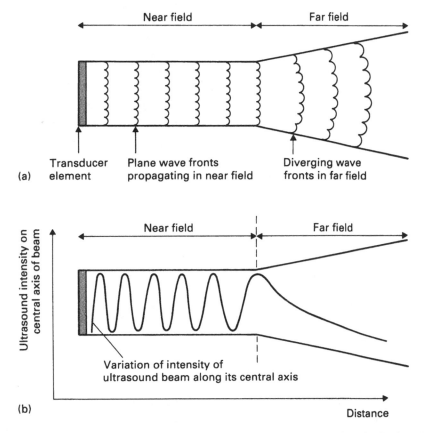

**Fig. 16.22** Ultrasound beam shape from a flat, circular transducer. (a) Longitudinal section through the centre of the beam; (b) intensity variation within the beam. The transducer element acts as if it were a large number of single, closely spaced ultrasound sources, each producing a single ultrasound wave. These individual waves interfere to produce a plane wave front and a complex intensity pattern within the beam. Note the regular intensity minima and maxima in the near field and the gradual reduction of intensity in the far field.

When the transducer element is pulsed, it acts as if it were a large number of single, closely spaced ultrasound sources each producing a single ultrasound wave (in accordance with Huygens' principle). These individual waves interfere to produce a plane wave front and a complex intensity pattern within the beam. The resultant ultrasound beam is initially cylindrical, beginning to diverge only after it has travelled some distance from the transducer element.

Within the **near field** (or Fresnel zone), the wave interference phenomenon persists and the plane wave front is maintained. The beam width in the near field is approximately the same as the transducer diameter.

In the **far field** (or Fraunhoffer zone), wave interference diminishes and the ultrasound beam begins to diverge, reducing rapidly in its intensity. The beam width in this part of the beam is increased.

The near field is *the most useful for imaging purposes*, as it is the narrowest part of the beam. It is, therefore, the part of the beam at which spatial resolution across the axis of the beam (lateral resolution) will be greatest. It is also the part of the beam in which intensity remains high, only reducing by approximately 5% along the length of the near field.

In the far field, energy is lost rapidly as the beam diverges. It thus significantly reduces the intensity of any reflected ultrasound and the likelihood of its reaching the transducer and being recorded as an echo. Lateral resolution is also poor, due to the increased beam width.

The length of the near field and the angle at which the far field diverges may be calculated as follows:

$$l = \frac{d^2}{4}$$

and

$$\sin \theta = \frac{1.22\lambda}{d}$$

where

| | | |
|---|---|---|
| $l$ | = | length of near field |
| $d$ | = | diameter of transducer element |
| $\lambda$ | = | wavelength of the ultrasound beam |
| $\sin \theta$ | = | sine of angle of divergence of far field |

It can be seen, therefore, that the diameter of the transducer element has a critical effect on the length of the near field. For a given wavelength of ultrasound: as the diameter of the transducer element increases so does the length of the near field of the ultrasound beam and, hence, its usefulness in ultrasound imaging. Unfortunately, as the diameter of the transducer element increases, lateral resolution reduces. In reality, therefore, the design diameter of a single element transducer is always a compromise between these factors depending largely upon the application for which the probe is designed.

### Shaped transducer elements

It is possible to change the shape of the ultrasound beam by shaping the transducer element so that it is concave. This has a focusing effect on the ultrasound beam, resulting in smaller beam width and greater intensity at the focal zone within the region that approximates to the near field. Beyond the focal zone, however, a penalty is experienced: the beam rapidly diverges from the focal zone – and while its width increases, its intensity decreases.

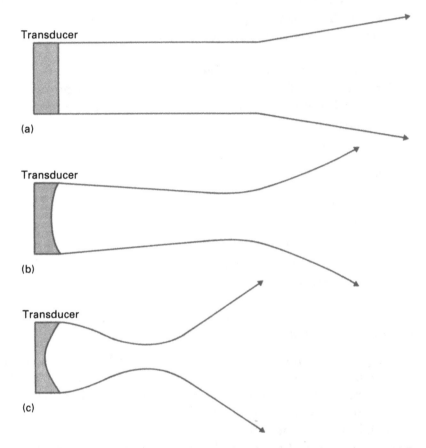

**Fig.16.23** The effect on the ultrasound beam of shaping the transducer element. (a) Beam shape from a flat transducer element; (b) beam shape from a moderately shaped element; (c) beam shape from a heavily shaped element. Shaping the transducer element so that it is concave has a focusing effect on the ultrasound beam, giving it reduced width and greater intensity at the focal zone within the region that approximates to the near field. Beyond the focal zone, however, width increases rapidly while beam intensity decreases.

### Thickness of the transducer element

The thickness of the transducer element is of fundamental importance to determining the operating frequency of the transducer. Operating frequency is determined by the relationship:

$$f_o = \frac{c_e}{2x}$$

where

$f_o$ = operating frequency of transducer
$c_e$ = speed of sound in transducer material
$x$ = required thickness of transducer element

The speed of sound for any given transducer element material is a constant. Thus, as the required operating frequency increases, the thickness of the transducer element used to produce a given frequency decreases.

### Thickness of the matching layer

The thickness of the matching layer is designed to provide maximum transmission of ultrasound from the matching layer to tissue. For a single matching layer:

$$T = \lambda/4$$

where

$T$ = thickness of the matching layer
$\lambda$ = wavelength of ultrasound in matching layer

A thickness of $\lambda/4$ produces ultrasound beam (signal) enhancement due to the way in which the propagating waves and the reflected waves constructively interfere.

### *Mechanical rotating and oscillating transducers*

Single-element transducers find their most common application in modern ultrasound imaging equipment, in the production of real time ultrasound images: mounted in mechanical rotating or oscillating devices which are moved rapidly so that a real time sector scanning action can be produced and, hence, a sector scan image.

The simpler of these two devices is the mechanical oscillating device. Within this, a single element transducer is made to pivot around a point. Within the constraints of the construction of the ultrasound probe, this point is positioned as close as possible to the centre of the front face of the transducer.

A mechanical rotating device, in its simplest form, is a wheel on which a single-element transducer is mounted so that the ultrasound beam is directed radially away from the centre of the wheel. It is usual, however, for three or four identical single-element transducers to be mounted on the wheel at equal spacings.

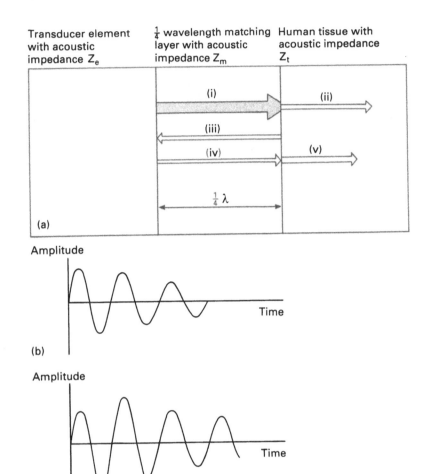

**Fig. 16.24** Matching layer thickness and signal intensity. (a) Schematic diagram showing transducer element, matching layer and tissue volume, with ultrasound waves at five stages.

*Key:*
Ultrasound waves:
(i)   Initially emitted by the transducer.
(ii)  Transmitted into the tissue, see (b).
(iii) Reflected at the interface between matching layer and tissue.
(iv)  Reflected again, at the interface between matching layer and transducer element.
(v)   Transmitted into the tissue with increased amplitude due to constructive interface between the ultrasound wave that was reflected at matching layer/transducer element interface and new ultrasound wavefront propagating from transducer element.

(b) Graphical representation of ultrasound transmitted into tissue (see (ii)). (c) Graphical representation of ultrasound entering tissue with increased amplitude due to constructive ultrasound wave interference (see (v)).

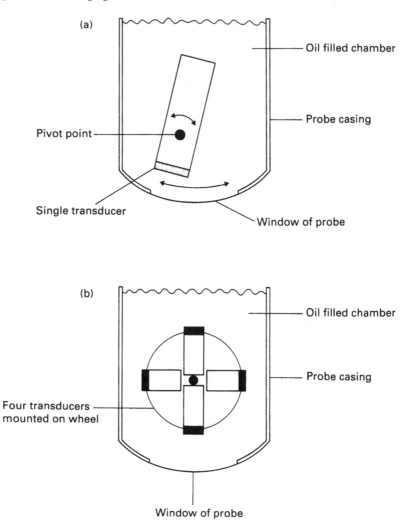

**Fig. 16.25** Schematic diagrams of (a) mechanical oscillating, and (b) mechanical rotating transducer.

In their construction, these two types of mechanically moved transducers have similarities: they are both contained within an **oil-filled housing**, the front face of which (usually a thin plastic membrane) is in intimate contact with human tissue during scanning. This arrangement ensures that the active transducer, immediately behind the front face, is positioned as close as possible to the skin surface.

A **drive or movement mechanism** is required in both, to rotate or pivot the transducer. Drive mechanisms may be either **direct** or **indirect**. In direct systems, a small electric motor drives a mechanical link attached either to the pivoted transducer or to the wheel on which the transducers are mounted. The indirect system involves a magnetic linkage between the drive motor and the rotating wheel or pivoting transducer. The indirect method is often preferred as it enables the whole of the transducer assembly and the drive mechanism to be contained within the oil-filled housing. This may also enable the probe to be made relatively small and lightweight.

It is important in relation to these transducers, that the relative position of the ultrasound beam at any point in time can be determined. This may be achieved in a number of ways although the principle of the various methods is common: essentially, it involves a friction-free magnetic device which is able to measure angles without direct contact between the moving parts.

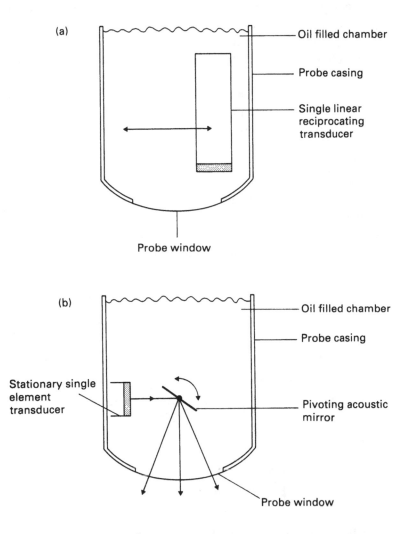

**Fig. 16.26** Schematic representation of (a) linear reciprocating, and (b) oscillating acoustic mirror transducers. These are two uncommon methods of using single-element transducers to produce real time ultrasound scanning.

Although uncommon, there are two further methods of using single-element transducers to produce real time ultrasound scanning:

(1) A linear, reciprocating single-element transducer; and
(2) A stationary, single-element transducer, used in conjunction with a pivoting acoustic mirror.

### Multi-element transducers

A large number of modern, real time ultrasound imaging systems use multi-element probes. These may be classic, **linear array** (or stepped array) probes, **curvilinear array** probes or **phased array** (electronically-steered array) probes. Probes with **annular array** transducers are also available, although these are found most commonly in mechanically oscillating transducer scanners.

In their construction and inherent beam-forming or beam-shaping principles, multi-element transducers are very similar to single-element transducers. They may, in fact, be considered to be a series of closely spaced, single-element transducers. Apart from annular-array transducers (which are composed of concentric rings of piezoelectric ceramic), the elements in multi-element transducers are rectangular in shape.

In the linear and curvilinear array transducers, small, overlapping groups of piezoelectric elements are pulsed sequentially. When fired, each group of elements contributes one line of information to the image. The sequential firing of groups of elements thus enables a complete image to be con-

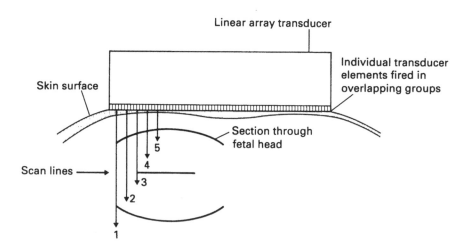

**Fig. 16.27** Image formation from a linear array transducer. Rapid, repeated, sequential firing of overlapping groups of elements, together with computer-driven control and manipulation, enables real time images to be produced: elements 1–5 produce scan line 1; 4–8 produce scan line 2; 7–11 produce line 3, and so on.

structed. Rapid repetition of this sequential firing, together with computer-driven control and manipulation components within the ultrasound scanner, enables real time ultrasound images to be produced.

In their requirements for matching layers, backing materials, electrodes and casings, multi-element transducers have similar requirements to single-element transducers. Their operating frequencies are governed by the thickness of the transducer element and the particular material of which it is made. Multi-element transducers differ however, in the machining of the transducer material and the focusing of the ultrasound beam which is under electronic control.

### Linear and curvilinear arrays

Electronic linear and curvilinear (curved) arrays are constructed and operated similarly, the single difference being the shape of the array.

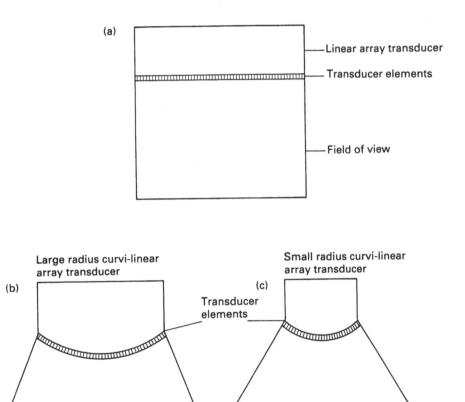

**Fig. 16.28** Fields of view from typical linear (a) and curved array transducers; large radius (b) and small radius (c). The relationship is shown between length of array and field of view.

Linear array transducers have a field of view that corresponds to the physical length of the array. In practice, this means that the field of view is limited and, if the array is short, may be insufficient to meet clinical imaging needs. If the length of the array is increased to provide a larger, more adequate field of view, however, difficulty may be experienced in maintaining intimate contact between the transducer and the surface of the body.

Curved array transducers overcome this problem, providing a relatively large field of view (particularly at depth within tissue) compared to their physical dimensions. As the radius of curvature decreases (i.e. the array is curved more acutely), the ratio of field of view to the physical dimensions of the transducer increases.

Typically, linear array transducers are used for abdominal ultrasound imaging and operate at 3.5 MHz. Such a transducer may contain 120 closely spaced but acoustically isolated piezoelectric elements, each approximately 10 mm × 1 mm. Some linear array transducers, however, are designed to operate at frequencies up to 10 MHz, and may have as few as 50 or as many as 400 elements. It should be remembered that, as with single-element transducers, the physical dimensions of the elements are determined by the

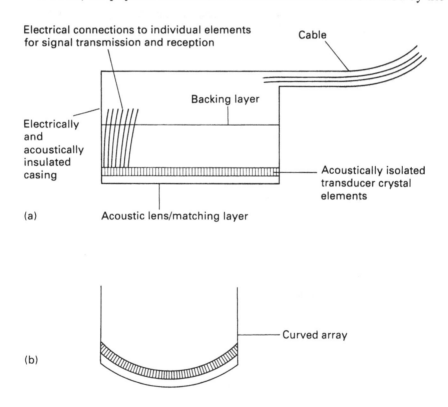

Fig. 16.29 Principles of construction of electronic transducers. (a) Linear array; (b) curved array (only differing from the linear array in that the crystal array is curved along its length).

required frequency of ultrasound. As the required frequency increases, the dimensions of the elements reduce.

Curved array transducers have a wide range of applications and are rapidly taking over the role of linear array transducers in abdominal imaging. They are very similar in construction to the linear arrays but tend to have fewer piezoelectric elements, particularly as their radius of curvature decreases (i.e. as they become more acutely curved). Typically, a transducer with a radius of curvature of 25 mm (sharply curved), operating at 3.5 MHz, will contain 50 piezoelectric elements.

The requirement for multi-element transducers to be composed of small, closely spaced but acoustically isolated piezoelectric elements may be achieved in one of two ways. Most commonly, a linear array transducer is formed by a precision machining process: parallel grooves are cut into a slab of piezoelectric ceramic whose overall size equals the required physical dimensions of the transducer. It is also possible, however, to construct a linear array transducer from completely separate, identical piezoelectric elements.

The major difference between single- and multi-element transducers lies in the electronic control of ultrasound beam focusing. It was noted pre-

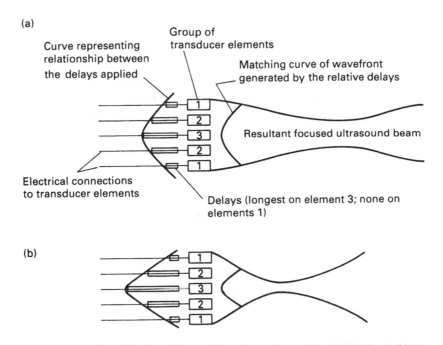

**Fig. 16.30** Principles of focusing electronic array transducers: (a) moderate focus; (b) strong focus. The delays on elements 2 and 3 are greater in the strong focus transducer. This generates a more sharply curved wavefront, increased focusing of the beam, and a focal zone closer to the group of elements.

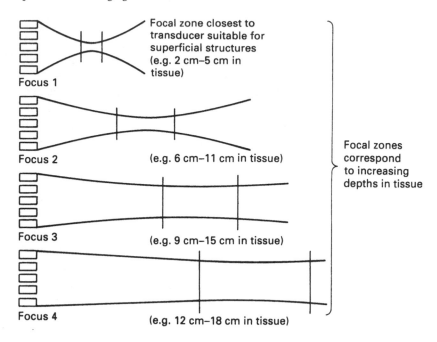

Focal zone closest to
transducer suitable for
superficial structures
(e.g. 2 cm–5 cm in
tissue)

Focus 1

Focus 2        (e.g. 6 cm–11 cm in tissue)

Focus 3        (e.g. 9 cm–15 cm in tissue)

Focus 4        (e.g. 12 cm–18 cm in tissue)

Focal zones
correspond
to increasing
depths in tissue

**Fig. 16.31** Variable electronic focusing from array transducers. The focus may be selected such that the focal zone (narrowest part) of the ultrasound beam can be made to coincide with the depth in tissue of the structures of most interest.

viously that a group of elements in an array transducer is fired to produce a single line of information in the ultrasound image. If all the elements within that group were to be fired simultaneously, they would act simply as a single-element, unfocused transducer. Instead, the firing sequence is such that the outer elements of the group are fired fractionally ahead of the inner elements, and the resulting ultrasound beam is focused.

This introduction of a time delay into the firing sequence of individual elements within a group produces a corresponding delay in the generation of the ultrasound wavefront and, hence, a focusing effect within the ultrasound beam. The degree to which the beam is focused depends upon the time delay between the firing of the outer elements and inner elements within a group. A *longer time delay* results in a *more highly focused* ultrasound beam. Ultrasound scanners are now equipped with controls which enable the focus of the ultrasound beam to be varied such that the narrowest part of the ultrasound beam can be made to coincide with those structures of most interest during an ultrasound imaging investigation.

**Multiple zone focusing** of the transmitted ultrasound beam is also possible. This is achieved by firing the same group of elements more than once, but with different time delays between the firing of the individual

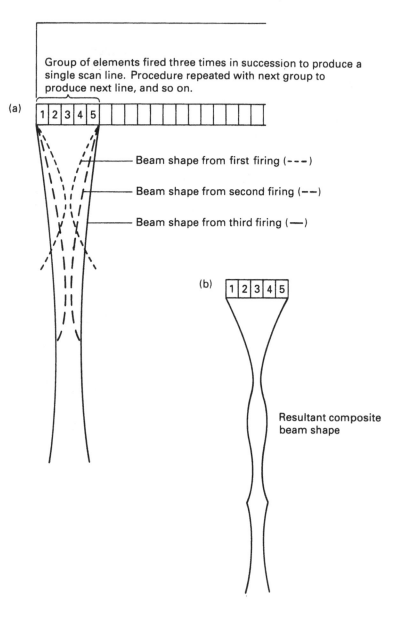

Fig. 16.32 Multiple zone focusing in transmission: (a) schematic representation of successive firing; (b) resultant composite beam shape. Different time delays are employed between the firing of individual elements within a group. The composite has more than one focal zone, making it narrow over a greater distance than would be the case if the group of elements were only fired once.

elements in the group. This produces a single scan line with more than one focal zone so that the effective ultrasound beam shape is made relatively narrow through a *greater distance* than would be the case if the group of elements were only fired once.

Multiple zone focusing in transmission increases ultrasound image resolution, but it is not without its problems. In particular, there is a reduction in the speed at which an ultrasound image is built up, since each scan line contributing to the image is formed from two, three or four sequential firings of each group of elements.

Associated with electronic focusing of the transmitted ultrasound beam (particularly in multiple zone focusing) is dynamic focusing *in reception*, i.e. of the beam reflected from tissues, back to the transducer.

This process requires electronic time delays to be applied to the echo signals generated at each transducer element. These are applied so that the

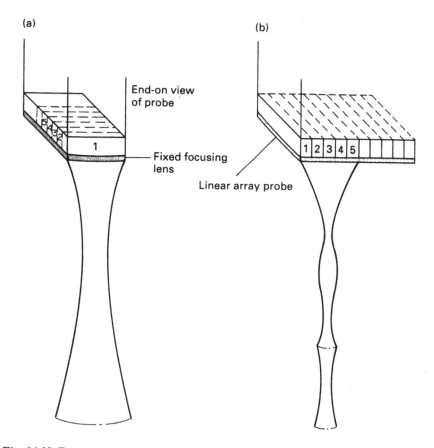

**Fig. 16.33** Focusing of an electronic linear array transducer. The contrast is shown between ultrasound beam shapes: (a) in the out-of-scan plane, due to use of a fixed focusing lens; and (b) in the scan plane, due to multiple zone electronic focusing.

reception focal zone corresponds to the depth in tissue from which the echoes arose.

The reception focal zone may be *swept* along the beam axis so that dynamic focusing is possible throughout the depth of tissue from which useful echoes are being received.

Electronic focusing of the ultrasound beam from a linear or curvilinear array transducer *is effective in one plane only*. This plane, often referred to as the **scan plane**, *lies at right angles to the long axis of the individual transducer elements*. It is possible to focus the ultrasound beam in the opposing plane, but only by attaching an ultrasound focusing lens to the front face of the transducer. Focusing in the out-of-scan plane is therefore fixed during the manufacturing process and cannot subsequently be altered.

An annular array transducer produces a *cylindrical* wave front. With such a transducer, it is possible to focus the ultrasound beam electronically and to maintain its cylindrical shape. Focusing of an annular array transducer is carried out by firing the outermost ring of piezoelectric elements first and the innermost ring last. Equal time delays are introduced between the firing of each of the rings so that equivalent time delays are introduced into the wave front. The resultant cylindrical ultrasound beam is, therefore, effectively narrowed, or focused. As the time delays are increased, so is the narrowing of the resultant ultrasound beam. Typically, an annular array transducer contains four or more concentric rings of piezoelectric elements.

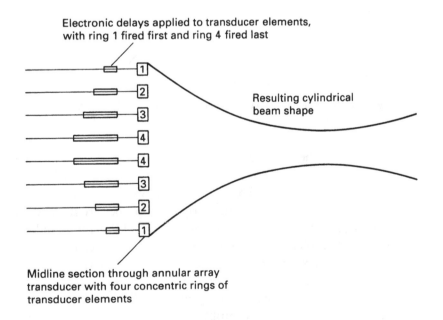

Fig. 16.34 Electronic focusing of an annular array transducer.

## Electronically steered (phased) arrays

Electronically steered array transducers are very similar in construction to linear array transducers. In size, steered arrays are much smaller, however, and contain fewer piezoelectric elements in their arrays. Typically, the faces of these probes are almost square in shape, measuring between 20 mm$^2$ and 40 mm$^2$. The number of elements varies between 20 and 120, depending upon the application for which a particular probe has been designed.

Steered array probes have been the natural choice for ultrasound imaging of the heart, as they have a number of features which particularly suit this application:

(1)  They are small and so allow an inter-costal approach to the heart.
(2)  From a small contact area, they have a wide sector angle or field of view – up to 90°.
(3)  They are relatively lightweight and thus easy to manoeuvre.

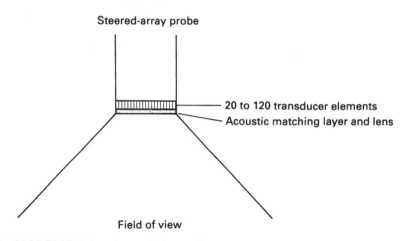

Steered-array probe

20 to 120 transducer elements
Acoustic matching layer and lens

Field of view

**Fig. 16.35** Field of view for a typical steered array probe. From a small contact area, steered array probes have a wide sector angle or field of view – up to 90°.

Control of the ultrasound beam shape is complex, however, and it is not easy to ensure that the characteristics of the ultrasound beam shape are similar throughout the whole of the sector sweep. Image quality can be less than optimum, therefore, particularly when probes are designed with large sector angles. Sophisticated computer control of the ultrasound beam shape from such probes has improved their performance, however, and with further development may make them more generally acceptable across a much broader range of ultrasound imaging applications.

Unlike linear and curved array probes, all piezoelectric elements in a steered array transducer contribute to each line of the ultrasound image. Their operation involves the introduction of delays into the firing sequence

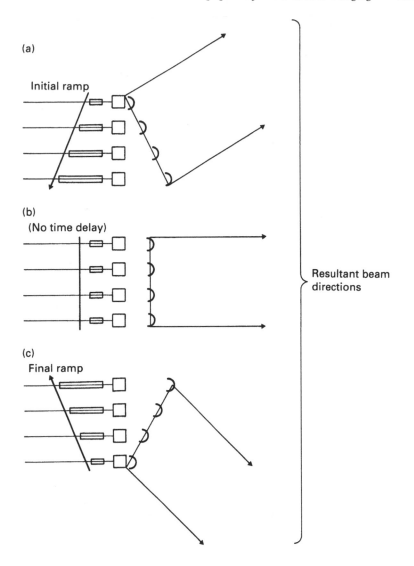

**Fig. 16.36** The principles of ultrasound beam steering in a steered array transducer. (a) Initial time delay ramp applied to firing of transducer elements; (b) no time delay applied; (c) final time delay ramp applied to firing of transducer elements.

of the elements so that the beam is, firstly, steered and, secondly, electronically focused.

Ultrasound beam steering is achieved by applying a **time delay ramp** across the firing of the transducer elements. This introduces a corresponding time delay ramp into the ultrasound wave front generated by the transducer. The resultant wave front, therefore, emerges from the transducer *at an angle to its face*. A change in the time delay ramp applied to the firing of the transducer elements will change the time delay ramp across the emerging ultrasound wave front and, hence, the angle between the wave front and the face of the transducer.

In order to produce a complete sector, the transducer elements are fired initially with a time delay ramp that produces the minimum required angle of the ultrasound beam to the transducer (i.e. it forms an acute angle with the transducer face). Subsequent time delay ramps are progressively decreased so that the scan lines form increasingly larger (less acute) angles with the transducer. When the time delay ramp reaches zero (i.e. when all elements are fired simultaneously), the ultrasound beam (and scan line) emerges at right angles to the front face of the transducer. At this point, half of the sector has been produced. To complete the sector, a gradually increasing time delay ramp is applied to the firing of the crystals. The

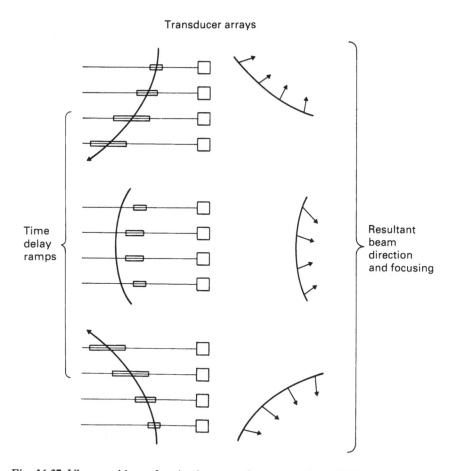

**Fig. 16.37** Ultrasound beam focusing in a steered array transducer. This illustrates the focusing effect on the ultrasound beam of applying non-linear time delay ramps to the firing of the transducer elements. The three examples show how the ramps can control both steering and focusing of the ultrasound beam.

ultrasound beams produced thus form decreasing angles, until the final scan line is produced with, again, the minimum required angle between the ultrasound beam and the front face of the transducer. Clearly, the time delay ramps applied to the firing of the elements at the extremes of the sector, though equal in time, are opposite in the direction in which they are applied to the transducer elements.

As with the linear and curved array transducers, it is also possible to focus steered array transducers in the scan plane. Again, however, focusing in the out-of-scan plane is only possible by the addition of a focusing lens to the front face of the transducer during manufacture.

Electronic focusing of steered array transducers in the scan plane is achieved by altering the shape of the time delay ramps which are applied to the firing of the transducer elements in order to steer the beam. Beam steering alone requires a linear time delay ramp to be applied. The combination of beam steering and beam focusing, however, requires the application of a non-linear time delay ramp.

## 16.8 B-mode, real time, grey scale ultrasound imaging systems

### Introduction

Real time, B-mode scanners are the most commonly used ultrasound equipment, producing real time, grey scale images. B-scanners range from hand-held portable units, through a range of machines that may be trans-

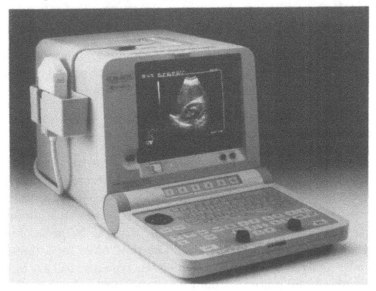

**Fig. 16.38** A portable, real time, grey scale B-scanner. (*The Hitachi EUB-405, courtesy of Diasonics Sonotron.*)

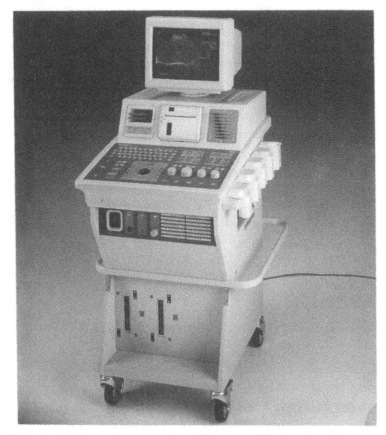

**Fig. 16.39** A typical, large, department based B-scanner. (*The Combison 410, courtesy of Kretztechnik UK Ltd.*)

ported on trolleys, to large machines with integral transport systems. These largest machines can be moved within a hospital but tend to be confined to a specific location, usually the ultrasound department.

### Real time scanning

In pulse-echo imaging, once a pulse of ultrasound has been produced by the transducer, it is necessary for the transducer to receive the resultant reflections (or echoes) before generating a second. Real time ultrasound imaging is possible because of the high speed at which ultrasound propagates in tissue (1540 ms$^{-1}$) and the fact that a single pulse of ultrasound is generated in approximately 1 μs. The time taken for a single episode of pulse generation and echo reception is, typically, 250 μs. In one second, therefore, the process of pulse generation and echo reception will occur 4000 times. Hence, 4000 lines of echo information will be collected in one second. A B-mode image is formed from sequential lines of information.

While real time B-scanners can generate images (or frames) at rates between 5 per second and 40 per second, a typical B-scanner using a 3.5 MHz transducer will generate images at a rate of *25 per second*, hence enabling tissue movement to be observed and the label *real time* to be applied. If a B-scanner is to produce images at a rate of 25 per second, when the process of pulse generation and echo reception occurs 4000 times in one second (number of lines per image = number of lines per second/number of images per second), it can be seen that each image will contain 160 lines of echo information.

In practice, the number of images per second (frame rate), the number of lines per image (line density) and the frequency and type of the transducer are interdependent. Reference to manufacturers' data supplied with their equipment, illustrates this.

**Table 16.3** Typical specifications of a real time, B-scanner, showing probe type, frequency, frame rate and line density. (*Compiled from data supplied with the Siemens Sonoline S1–250, courtesy of Siemens plc.*)

| Probe type | Frequency (MHz) | Frame rate (per second) | Line density |
|---|---|---|---|
| Linear array | 3.5 | 24 | 113 |
| | 5.0 | 31 | 113 |
| Sector probe | 3.5 | 24 | 109 |
| | 5.0 | 30 | 109 |

## *Grey scale imaging*

In parallel with real time imaging, grey scale imaging has significantly increased the role of ultrasound in medical diagnosis. In particular, grey scale imaging in ultrasound has enabled tissue information from the vast number of weak echoes (those arising predominantly from scatter interactions) to be demonstrated in the ultrasound images.

The objective of grey scale imaging, described simply, is to represent the range of echo amplitudes received by the transducer as different shades of grey in the final, viewed image. The dynamic range of received echo amplitudes may be as much as 50 dB (i.e. with a ratio of the largest amplitude to the smallest of approximately 316:1). Some compression of this dynamic range, in the order of 30 dB (approximately 30:1) may take place, although this now occurs less frequently than in the past. Typically, modern, digital scan converters assign the range of received echo amplitudes across 256 grey levels, using an 8-bit computer memory – even though it is impossible for the human eye to distinguish this number of grey shades in an image.

All modern ultrasound imaging units use sophisticated computers to achieve grey scale imaging. Each equipment manufacturer will offer particular features related to grey scale imaging which, in its opinion, are beneficial to image quality. The basic functions of these computers, however, remain similar.

A component within the signal manipulation and storage core module, which controls signal digitization and storage, enables grey scale imaging to

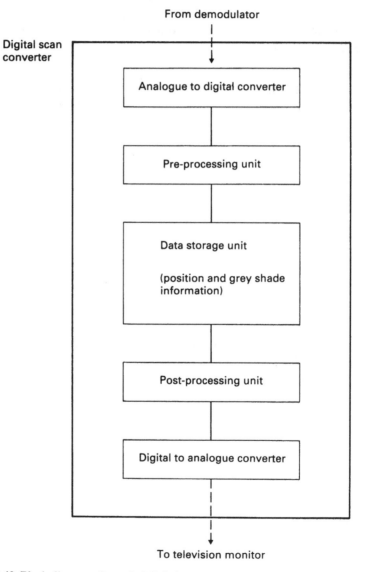

Fig. 16.40 Block diagram of a typical digital scan converter.

take place. This component is most commonly referred to as the **digital scan converter**.

### Digital scan converters

Digital scan converters are computers that store echo information, typically in an 8-bit matrix of digital memory elements, or pixels. Initially, the digital scan converter receives echo information in the form of an analogue voltage signal (the smooth, envelope output from the demodulator). This signal is sampled at closely spaced, regular intervals and digitized, or assigned numerical values using binary notation, prior to storage. These binary numbers are stored in the digital memory elements and represent both the grey shades that correspond to the received echo amplitudes and the position from which those echoes arose in the body.

During storage of the digital signal, the signal compression referred to earlier may also take place. If present, such pre-processing will act to preserve most appropriately the useful diagnostic information received and, in particular, will act to preserve the weaker echoes.

Once the initial echo information has been stored in the computer memory, it will need updating regularly as successive lines of echo information are generated. A variety of approaches to updating stored information – updating algorithms – are available, of which two are used most widely. One simply replaces old information for new; hence the ultrasound image is continuously renewed as the tissue or structure under examination is scanned. The second replaces old information with a value which is the average of the old and the new values. Practically, this second approach has no effect on the speed at which images are generated and may produce a more accurate representation of the relative reflective characteristics of the tissues within an image.

The stored digital signals are unsuitable for display as a visual image and it is necessary for them to be converted to an analogue (voltage) signal. Prior to this conversion process, it is usual to manipulate the stored signals so that the image may be displayed with different contrast ranges. This is carried out without affecting the original stored echo data and, hence, it is possible to display an image with a contrast range other than the *standard* without losing any of the stored data. Three major post-processing options exist which allow:

(1) Compression of the low level signals;
(2) Compression of the high level signals; or
(3) Compression of both the low and high level signals so displaying preferentially the midrange signals.

Once post-processing is complete, it is necessary to produce a visible image. Invariably, this appears on a television display screen. The digital-to-

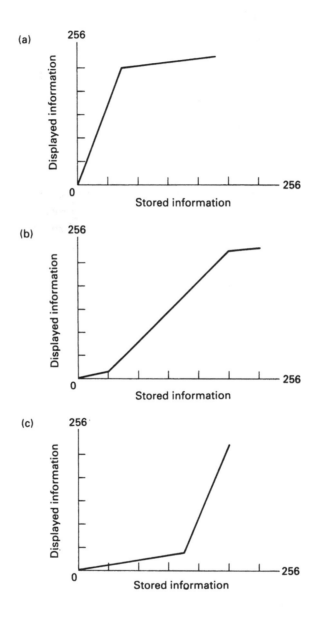

**Fig. 16.41** Post-processing signal manipulations. Three major post-processing options are shown: (a) Preferential display of low amplitude echo information, with compression of high amplitude echoes. (b) Preferential display of mid-range echoes, with some compression of both high and low amplitude echoes. (c) Preferential display of high amplitude echoes, with compression of low amplitude echoes.

analogue converter within the scan converter now acts to convert each binary digit stored in the memory into an analogue signal in the form of a voltage pulse. The amplitudes of these voltage pulses correspond to the values of the stored binary digits which represent particular grey shades, corresponding to amplitudes of the original received echoes. The voltage pulses form the video signal to the television display, where they control the intensity of the electron beam as it scans the television tube phosphor and, hence, the brightness (or grey scale) of the television image.

As well as grey scale, it is important that information about the positions within the tissue from which echoes arise is reproduced accurately on the television display. To achieve this, the computer matrix memory is scanned or *written out* line by line and is synchronized with the raster scan action of the electron beam. Complete images (or frames) are displayed at the rate of approximately 25 per second to give flicker-free viewing of images.

## Features of real time, grey scale B-scanning units

The computer technology which controls modern ultrasound equipment enables manufacturers to offer a wide variety of additional features on their ultrasound machines. Some features are claimed to be unique – for example, the introduction of three-dimensional imaging – while others are common to the majority of manufacturers. Students are recommended to obtain and analyse a range of manufacturers' technical specification sheets, as an exercise in the identification of the common features.

Mention of the full range of possible features is beyond the scope of this chapter. However, there are some of such importance that they must now be considered as standard features of all real time, grey scale B-scanning equipment.

### Choice of ultrasound probes, scanning methods and display modes
All real time, grey scale B-scanners, except those that are strictly portable, are equipped with a variety of ultrasound probes and enable ultrasound imaging in at least two modes.

### Time or depth–gain compensation
An essential feature of all B-scanners is time or depth–gain compensation applied to the voltage signals generated at the transducer by the received echoes.

A variety of methods enabling the operator to control time–gain compensation (TGC) are available. A simple system includes two controls. These (a) set the initial level at which TGC is applied (often referred to as the near-gain control) and (b) set the rate of increase of gain (the slope or far-gain). This system often includes a modification which forms a third

**Table 16.4** Typical combination of scanning probes and display modes. (*Data refer to the Toshiba Sonolayer SSA-250A, courtesy of Toshiba Medical Systems Ltd.*)

| Scanning probes | Display modes |
| --- | --- |
| Electronic convex | B-mode |
| Electronic linear | M-mode (including simultaneous B/M) |
| Electronic sector | |
| | Doppler mode (optional) |
| Mechanical sector | |
| Annular array sector | |

control, known as the TGC delay. This delays the application of increasing gain (the slope) for a short period.

A more sophisticated system uses a series of slider controls such that each applies TGC to those echoes that arise from a specific depth range within the tissue. Typically, the depth range of the machine (which corresponds to the depth of tissue to be scanned) is divided into 2 cm segments. The slider control for each segment applies the appropriate TGC for that segment according to the type of echoes being generated from the corresponding tissue depth. These controls enable weak echoes to receive high gain and strong echoes to receive low gain, irrespective of the depth from which they arise.

As TGC is controlled by the operator, it is important that there is a visual display of the TGC being applied. The display may be graphical or numerical data shown alongside the image, or by reference to calibrated controls on the control panel.

Some manufacturers offer automated TGC function. This is controversial, however, and it is rare that automated TGC is offered exclusively.

## Beam focusing in transmission and receive modes

Ultrasound beam focusing during transmission of the ultrasound beam into tissue (multiple zone focusing) and dynamic focusing of the returning ultrasound beam were discussed earlier. Nevertheless, it is of such fundamental importance within ultrasound equipment that it is necessary to refer to it again. As was mentioned, beam focusing is achieved in the scan plane by electronic means, through the use of sophisticated computer systems. Considerable efforts are made by manufacturers to improve their electronic beam focusing systems, in both transmission and receive modes, as these features are central to the image resolution, particularly lateral resolution, that may be achieved. As lateral resolution is the principal factor governing

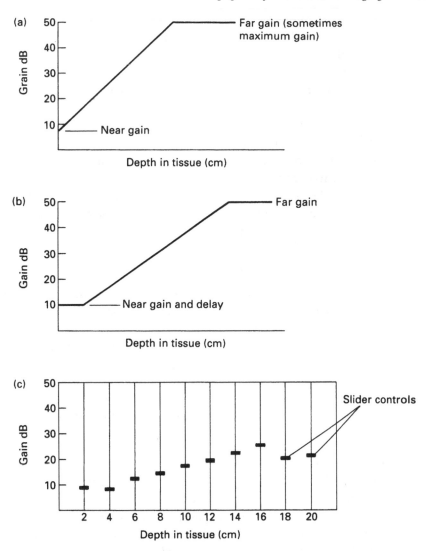

Fig. 16.42 Time–gain compensation systems. (a) Simple, two–control system (near and far gain controls): the two controls together determine the rate of increase of gain (i.e. the slope). (b) Simple, three–control system (near gain, far gain and delay controls). (c) Complex, slider controls system. The controls can be varied considerably, independently of each other.

the detail recognizable in an ultrasound image, it is apparent that the degree and quality of beam focusing will determine the amount of detail which can be distinguished in an image.

Reference to manufacturers' technical data reveals a considerable variety of options for multiple zone focusing in transmission, and for dynamic focusing in reception. Some ultrasound machines, typically those at the bottom end of the price spectrum, have only one or two transmission focal zone settings. Other machines at the top end of the range may have as many as seven. Typically, however, a machine will have four transmission focal zone settings, two or three of which will be used for most general scanning applications.

Similarly, there are considerable differences in the technical specifications of the dynamic focusing in reception features. Such features may be *dynamic* but, in reality, consist of eight focusing zones or may be continuous, varying from 0.5 cm to 24 cm.

One limitation of beam focusing is the dependence on physical methods (lens systems) for focusing in the out-of-scan plane. This is likely to be overcome shortly, however, so that electronic focusing systems which enable focusing in both the scan and the out-of-scan planes will become features of ultrasound equipment.

## Pre-processing and post-processing options

These have been discussed previously. Nevertheless, it is important to recognize that all manufacturers offer these options. More importantly, it is vital that the users of ultrasound machines recognize the need to familiarize themselves with these features in the context of their clinical work. It may, for example, be useful to use the post-processing function to increase the contrast in the viewed image when examining small cystic structures embedded in the substance of an organ. Such a decision, however, and similar decisions, must only be made when the effect of using post-processing is fully understood.

### Image freeze

One essential feature of all ultrasound machines is the feature enabling an image to be frozen on the screen. This permits close scrutiny of a structure to take place without further exposure to ultrasound energy. It also allows measurements to be made of structures within the image and facilitates down loading of selected images to hard-copy devices so that a permanent record of the image can be made.

### Magnification facility

A magnification facility enables scanning to take place of a small but enlarged part of a structure. While this can be useful, it tends to be limited by the resolution of the image; in particular, as magnification is increased, the pixels become evident.

### Electronic calipers

The electronic calipers, present on all machines, are a very important feature. Caliper functions available include measurement of distance, circumference, area and volume.

Electronic calipers must be calibrated to the correct speed of propagation of ultrasound in tissue which, for all general applications, is 1540 ms$^{-1}$.

Associated with the functioning of the electronic calipers may be a range of measurement software programs. These enable measurements obtained by the calipers to be translated into physiological or biological data. For example, a measurement of the crown–rump length of a fetus may be displayed not only as a distance measurement, but also as gestational age in weeks and days.

### Image display manipulation

Images can be black/white reversed so that the operator can select whether to view positive or negative images. Right/left and top/bottom image reversal is also possible. The television screen may be divided so that two or four images can be displayed. Although only one of these images may be viewed dynamically, this facility does enable a structure to be examined in more than one plane, directly on the television screen.

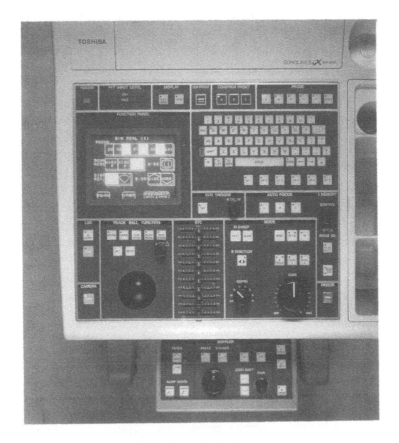

**Fig. 16.43** A typical control panel. (*The Toshiba Sonolayer SSA-250A, courtesy of Toshiba Medical Systems Ltd.*)

### Data display

It is also usual for image data to be displayed on the television screen. Some may be displayed automatically, while others are selected or entered by the user. Data displayed automatically include date, time, probe type and frequency, frame rate, focusing, TGC, power level, pre-processing option and post-processing option. Other data which may be entered by the user include patient information and body markers which indicate the location and plane of scan being carried out.

B-scanners feature an alphanumeric keyboard or touch pad which can be used to enter patient information, but which may also be used to annotate images as required. This may be useful for identifying pathology directly on an image or for teaching purposes.

### *Image display equipment*

Television monitors used in ultrasound imaging are constructed and operate as described in Chapter 7. Typically, 625 line, monochrome television monitors are used in ultrasound imaging, with screen sizes of 23 cm, 30 cm or 35 cm. The increase in colour Doppler applications, however, seems likely to make colour monitors the norm.

### Image recording in ultrasound

No real time, grey scale B-scanning unit is complete without at least one method of obtaining permanent hard copy images. The method (or methods) chosen for a particular machine will reflect both the purpose for which the machine was purchased and the projected costs of purchasing and running the chosen image recording system(s).

A large variety of image recording systems are available, varying enormously in both capital and running costs. These include dedicated, multi-imaging units which photograph images from a slave television monitor onto transparency film; video thermal imagers; optical laser disks; and videotape recorders.

A general purpose B-scanner, used for both abdominal and obstetric/gynaecological scanning, is likely to be equipped with two systems: a multi-imager or a laser imager, and a videotape recorder.

## 16.9 Doppler ultrasound

### *Introduction*

Continuous wave Doppler has been used for many years to study blood flow velocity in the body. Its limitation is that there is no provision of anatomical information. Doppler ultrasound has been revolutionized in recent years,

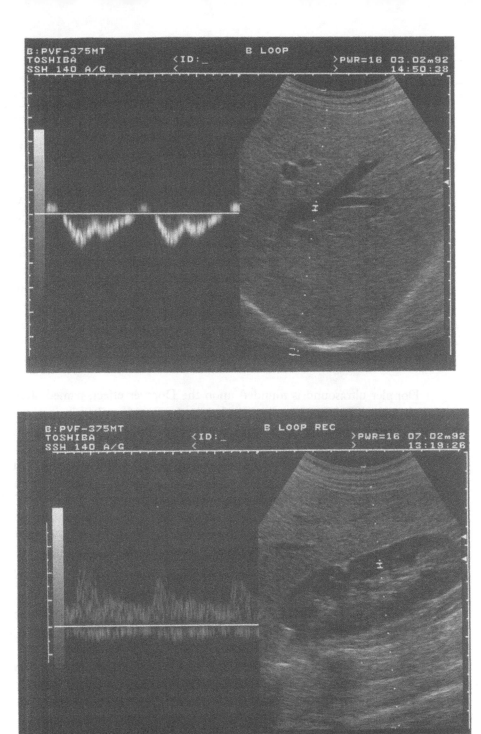

**Fig. 16.44** Simultaneous B–Mode and pulsed Doppler studies. (*Courtesy of Toshiba Medical Systems Ltd.*) Two examples of simultaneous B-mode/pulsed Doppler studies are shown. Note the *gate* within the hepatic vein in (a). Blood flow from this point in the hepatic vein is being explored using pulsed wave Doppler ultrasound and is giving rise to the Doppler spectrum shown alongside the image. (*By courtesy of Toshiba Medical Systems Ltd.*)

however, by technical advances, particularly in computer technology. Since the combination of simultaneous B-mode imaging and pulsed wave Doppler has been developed, the amount of information which can be obtained has increased significantly: high quality anatomical images acquired using B-mode ultrasound allow blood flow at specifically identified sites to be investigated using the Doppler mode.

Grey scale, simultaneous B-mode/Doppler imaging is still widely used, but it is being superseded by colour flow duplex imaging. This equipment provides colour coded Doppler data giving velocity information directly onto the B-mode images. A further advance is colour velocity imaging in which Doppler data, rather than being gathered separately, are obtained from the data contained in the image scan lines which form the B-mode image.

### Principles of Doppler ultrasound

Doppler ultrasound is founded upon the Doppler effect, named after the physicist, Christian Doppler (1803–53) who first described it.

The classic illustration of the Doppler effect involves a train approaching and leaving a station platform. In fact, early experimental work on the Doppler effect was based on just this situation. The pitch (frequency) of the noise made by the train appears higher as it approaches an observer on the station platform than when it is stationary at the platform. Similarly, as the train departs, the pitch of its noise as observed from the platform appears to be lower than when it was stationary.

The Doppler effect in ultrasound may be defined as a change in the observed frequency of an ultrasound wave when there is relative movement between the source of the ultrasound wave and the observer:

- When the motion of the source of the ultrasound wave is *towards* the observer, the observed frequency of the ultrasound wave is *higher* than if the ultrasound source were stationary.
- When the motion of the source of the ultrasound wave is *away from* the observer, the observed frequency of the ultrasound wave is *lower* than if that source were stationary.

In diagnostic medical applications of Doppler ultrasound, the original source of the ultrasound wave is the stationary transducer. The ultrasound beam produced at the transducer is directed towards a moving structure, for example a flow of blood cells. If the blood cells are moving in a direction which is towards the transducer, the transducer will perceive the frequency of the ultrasound reflected from them to be higher than the frequency of the transmitted ultrasound incident upon them. Equally, if blood cells are

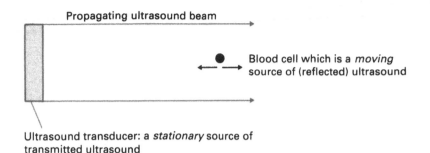

**Fig. 16.45** The principles of Doppler ultrasound. When the blood cell is moving *towards* the transducer, it reflects ultrasound (detected by the transducer) of a *higher* frequency than the original transmission. Moving *away from* the transducer, the blood cell reflects a *lower* frequency signal. Variations of frequency (compared with the original) are thus indicators of the blood cell's direction and rate of movement.

moving away from the transducer, the frequency of the reflected ultrasound as measured by the transducer will be lower than the frequency of the original, transmitted ultrasound. *The difference in magnitude* between the incident and reflected ultrasound frequencies is the **Doppler shift frequency**. For flowing blood, this has a value typically in the order of a few kilohertz and thus lies in the *audible sound* range.

There is a relationship between the speed of the moving structure and the resultant Doppler shift frequency. As the speed of movement increases, so too does the Doppler shift frequency. This relationship is shown quantitatively in the equations:

$$f_D = f_o - f_i$$

or

$$f_D = f_o\,(2\,\mu/c)$$

where

$f_D$ = Doppler shift frequency
$f_o$ = transmitted frequency
$f_i$ = reflected frequency
$\mu$ = speed of moving structure
$c$ = speed of ultrasound in tissue

In practical terms, it is necessary also to take into account the angle between the direction of the propagating ultrasound beam and the direction in which the moving structure is moving as shown in the formula below:

$$f_D = f_o\,(2\mu \cos\theta/c)$$

where $\cos\theta$ is the cosine of the angle between the propagating beam and the moving structure.

While Doppler ultrasound technology is complex, much of the complexity is associated with the analysis of echoes returning from the moving blood or whatever structure is being examined. The basic physical principles of Doppler ultrasound, as described, still apply.

## Equipment for Doppler ultrasound

Duplex ultrasound scanning equipment, in which real time B-scanning instruments are combined with Doppler facilities, is still a common provision. This equipment enables conventional, real time B-scanning to be performed, but also allows a Doppler dedicated ultrasound beam to address selected locations within the B-mode image, in order to analyse moving structures. In certain clinical applications, however – notably cardiac examinations – these conventional duplex systems are being displaced by equipment offering colour flow and colour velocity imaging.

Duplex systems may use mechanical sector probes, linear or curvilinear probes or phased-array probes, to generate B-mode images. Whatever the type of probe, an ultrasound beam position will be selected which will enable Doppler ultrasound data to be collected from the location specified on the B-mode image. During B-mode imaging, the site from which

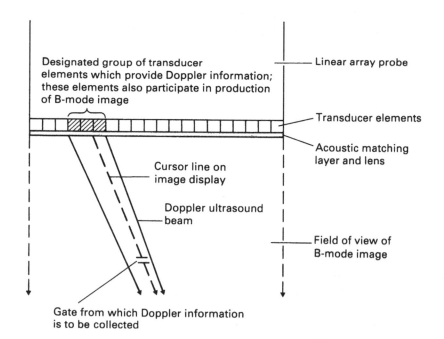

**Fig. 16.46** Linear-array probe in Doppler mode. In Doppler mode, a linear array probe uses a small group of elements fired in a sequence which directs (or steers) the ultrasound beam at an angle to the B-mode field, corresponding to the position of the electronic cursor.

Doppler information is to be collected is identified on the television monitor using an electronic cursor and gate. Doppler information is then collected, using one selected ultrasound beam positioned according to the electronic cursor.

In the case of a mechanical sector probe, the selected ultrasound beam will be the one produced at the particular angular position of the probe corresponding to the position of the electronic cursor.

Linear-array probes use a small group of elements fired in a sequence which directs (or steers) the ultrasound beam at an angle to the B-mode image and which corresponds to the position of the electronic cursor. Phased-array probes, like linear-array probes, also steer the Doppler ultrasound beam electronically to the required position.

Once the Doppler mode has been engaged, the equipment functions such that both the B-mode real time image and the Doppler information displayed are updated regularly. The Doppler information is updated preferentially and almost continuously, but the B-mode image is only updated with new information at intervals of approximately 1 second. These large intervals are not usually apparent to the operator, because the digital scan converter enables a real time image (although composed of *old* information) to be displayed.

## 16.10  Safety in ultrasound

Hazards to patients from the use of diagnostic medical ultrasound equipment may arise from a number of sources. These include:

(1) Deleterious biological effects from the ultrasound energy.
(2) Local heating of tissue in contact with probe, in which there is significant electrical heating during operation.
(3) The possibility of electric shock, if shock-proofing becomes compromised.
(4) Inadequately trained operators who do not understand the physical principles of ultrasound imaging and, hence, either fail to demonstrate significant abnormalities, or depict normal structures as abnormal.

Of these, the biological effects and operator error are the most important.

### *Biological effects of diagnostic ultrasound*

Considerable research into the biological effects of ultrasound has been carried out, although only a small proportion of this work has been directed at *in vivo* studies with diagnostic ultrasound.

The general conclusion drawn from the research is that, at the ultrasound intensities used in diagnostic medical ultrasound, no adverse effects on mammalian tissue have been confirmed. While this is accepted, it is important, for the following reasons, that exposure to ultrasound be minimized at all times.

Firstly, certain specialist applications (particularly some cardiac, neurological and transvaginal ultrasound investigations), as well as some of the recent highly sophisticated ultrasound units, use ultrasound intensities that are above the maximum recommended limit of $100\,\mathrm{mWcm}^{-2}$ (power). This figure is derived from statements on safety issued by the American Institute for Ultrasound in Medicine in 1987 (Bioeffects considerations for the safety of diagnostic ultrasound, *J. Ultrasound Med.*, 7, No. 9, supplement). It is the intensity below which no adverse biological effects have been confirmed using diagnostic ultrasound equipment (i.e. equipment using frequencies in the diagnostic range).

Secondly, it may be difficult to determine the power output of any particular ultrasound machine as there is little uniformity in the way this information is presented by manufacturers. It is also difficult to measure in a clinical ultrasound department and requires highly specialized, expensive test equipment.

Finally, the range of applications for which diagnostic ultrasound is being used is increasing considerably, as is the number of ultrasound scans carried out. For example, three ultrasound scans may now be carried out as *routine* during pregnancy, whereas previously one ultrasound scan was the norm. Now also, one or more of the three scans may include a transvaginal or a Doppler examination.

### Exposure reduction

There are several ways in which the operator may minimize exposure of patients to ultrasound. These include:

(1) Carrying out ultrasound scans *only where there is likely to be a benefit to the patient* (i.e. justified by a risk/benefit analysis).
(2) Ensuring that equipment does not emit intensities greater than $100\,\mathrm{mWcm}^{-2}$.
(3) Using the *lowest possible transmitted power settings*.
(4) Applying high gain to the *reflected* ultrasound beam rather than high power to the transmitted beam, to improve the sensitivity of the unit (i.e. the ability of the system to detect weak echoes).
(5) *Minimizing the period of exposure* to ultrasound during every ultrasound examination.
(6) *Removing the probe from the skin surface* whenever possible, during scanning.

(7) Checking that the transducer *does not transmit ultrasound when the image is frozen.*

*Operator error*

It is a truism that ultrasound scanning is highly operator dependent. Operators must have a thorough knowledge of normal human anatomy and must understand the physical principles governing both interactions of ultrasound with tissue and formation of the ultrasound image. In particular, operators must recognize the potential for abnormalities to be masked or mimicked by the production of **artefacts** in an image.

Artefacts in ultrasound images are spurious echo patterns which do not represent accurately the anatomical structures being scanned. A large number of recognized artefacts may occur during ultrasound scanning and *mimic abnormality*. An example is a simple cyst which appears to contain echoes. These echoes may be artefact only or may represent an abnormal structure within the cyst and, hence, pathology. Less commonly, but no less importantly, *abnormalities may be masked* by artefact. For example, small but pathological changes in liver tissue may not be demonstrated in the ultrasound image if gain settings are incorrectly adjusted.

Artefacts in ultrasound imaging may be impossible to avoid and, indeed, some artefacts may be helpful to the operator. In any ultrasound examination, however, the operator must understand how all the artefacts which may be encountered are produced, so that they can be dealt with or used appropriately.

## 16.11 Care of ultrasound equipment

Ultrasound equipment, like all equipment used in diagnostic imaging, must be properly and regularly maintained if it is to function correctly. Within every ultrasound department, a **quality assurance programme**, including routine equipment maintenance and quality control tests, must be established.

Routine equipment maintenance must be sufficiently thorough to ensure that equipment is clean and electrically safe. It should also have the effect of preventing minor operational faults from occurring, by including checks that electrical connections are secure and by reducing the risk of damage to probes.

A daily maintenance programme might include the following:

(1) Thorough cleaning of the ultrasound scanner and all its probes.
(2) Checking the ultrasound probe cables to ensure they are intact and properly connected.

(3) Checking the ultrasound probe housing to ensure that it is undamaged.
(4) Checking the operation of the ultrasound scanner and its associated imaging equipment to ensure it is working, prior to scanning any patients.

In addition, care should be taken to ensure that acoustic coupling gel is removed from the probe following each patient and that the probe is replaced carefully in its cradle.

Ultrasound equipment must also be subject to regular, routine quality control tests, thoroughly documented with supporting images. As a minimum, these tests must include checks on sensitivity; dynamic range; axial, lateral and contrast resolution; and caliper accuracy. Proprietary test phantoms which enable these tests to be carried out are available and *should be in every ultrasound department*.

The frequency with which quality control tests should be carried out is a matter to be determined locally. It may vary according to a particular test: for example, caliper accuracy may be tested weekly, while sensitivity checks may be carried out at three monthly intervals. What is important, however, is the need to *establish and maintain a regular pattern of testing*.

## 16.12 Conclusion

It has been impossible to discuss all aspects of ultrasound equipment within this single chapter. Instead, there has been a concentration on the equipment which student radiographers are likely to encounter in clinical practice. Further reading is therefore recommended, in which the accompanying bibliography may be helpful.

## 16.13 Bibliography

Athey, P.A. & McClendon, I. (1983) *Diagnostic Ultrasound for Radiographers*. Multi-media Publishing, Chislehurst.

Evans, D.H. *et al.* (1989) *Doppler Ultrasound Physics, Instrumentation and Clinical Applications*. Wiley, New York.

Fish, P. (1990) *Physics and Instrumentation of Diagnostic Medical Ultrasound*. Wiley, New York.

Kremkau, F.W. (1989) *Diagnostic Ultrasound Principles, Instruments and Exercises*. W.B. Saunders, Philadelphia.

Lerski, R.A. (Ed.) (1988) *Practical Ultrasound*. IRL Press, Oxford.

McDicken, W.N. (1991) *Diagnostic Ultrasonics Principles and Use of Instruments*. Churchill Livingstone, Edinburgh.

Shirley, I.M. *et al.* (1978) *A User's Guide to Diagnostic Ultrasound.* Pitman Medical, London.

Taylor, K.J.W. (1978) *Atlas of Gray Scale Ultrasonography.* Churchill Livingstone, Edinburgh.

Webb, S. (Ed.) (1988) *The Physics of Medical Imaging.* Adam Hilger.

# Chapter 17
# Magnetic Resonance Imaging

## 17.1 Introduction

Magnetic resonance imaging (MRI) is a diagnostic technique which does not involve the use of ionizing radiations. Magnetic resonance images are constructed by computer from data collected during the process of nuclear magnetic resonance (NMR) examinations of the patient. It is from NMR that magnetic resonance imaging derives its name. NMR has been used in the spectroanalysis of small samples for over four decades. Since the mid 1970s, magnets have been developed which produce a suitably homogeneous field and are large enough for human subjects. A brief explanation of NMR is essential before the design and function of magnetic resonance scanners can be appreciated.

## 17.2 NMR

NMR analysis is used to determine the presence and concentration of certain atomic nuclei within a sample. When NMR is performed, the parameters of the experiment are set in order to single out a particular type of atomic nucleus for investigation. The resulting NMR signal originates only from within those atoms and is modified by their biochemical environment.

The hydrogen atom is the target for MRI because it is widely distributed throughout the body and gives a relatively strong signal. The simplicity of hydrogen also makes it a suitable model for this explanation.

### Nuclear magnetism

The nucleus of a hydrogen atom consists of a single spinning proton carrying a positive electrical charge. The rotation of its charge gives rise to a dipole magnetic field surrounding the proton. The central axis of this field coincides with the rotational axis of the proton. Normally, protons in the body tissues would be spinning with their axes pointing in random directions.

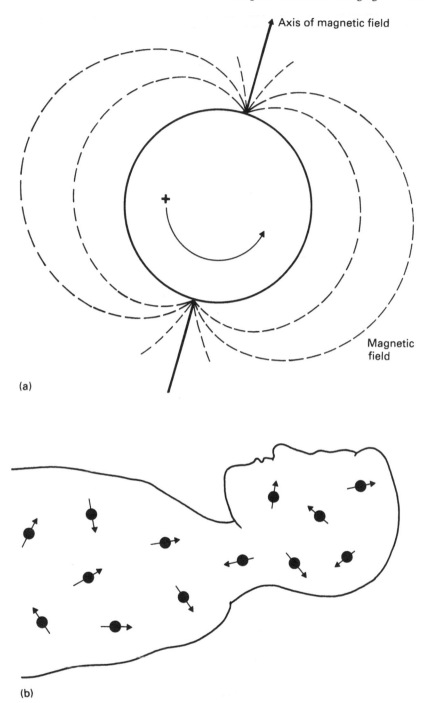

Axis of magnetic field

Magnetic field

(a)

(b)

**Fig. 17.1** Nuclear magnetism. (a) A spinning proton with its associated magnetic field. Rotation gives rise to a dipole magnetic field surrounding the proton. Its central axis coincides with the rotational axis of the proton, indicated by the arrow. (b) The normal, random orientation of proton spins throughout a patient.

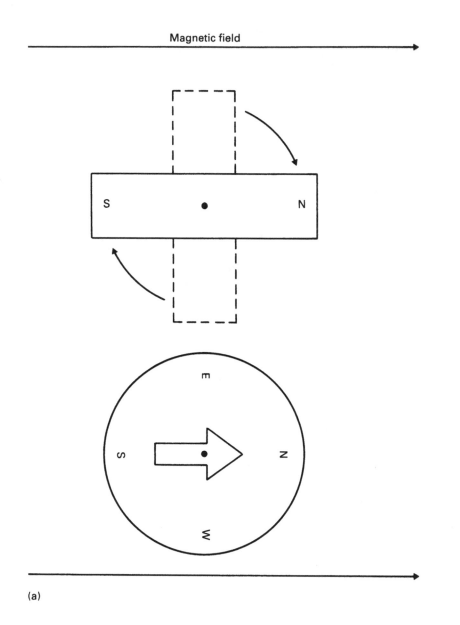

(a)

Fig. 17.2 Precession. (a) A freely suspended bar magnet and a magnetized compass needle orientate their axes parallel to an applied magnetic field. This is due to an interaction between the applied field and the field surrounding the magnetized object. (b) A spinning proton precessing in a magnetic field. A spinning proton also attempts to align its magnetic axis parallel to an external field. The proton spin creates an additional force which causes its axis to describe a circle around the direction in which it is pointing. This action is called precession.

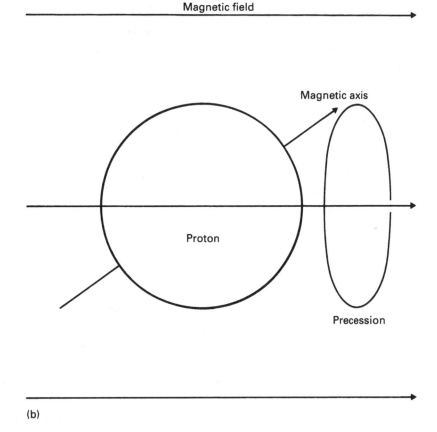

(b)

Other nuclei also possess magnetic fields and respond to NMR experiments. The presence of nuclear magnetism is determined by a factor related to the pairs of protons or neutrons in the nucleus. An uneven number of either particle will give rise to a magnetic field as the nucleus spins. For example:

*Carbon 12*: This common nuclide of carbon contains three pairs of protons and three pairs of neutrons. No magnetic field is produced by this combination and NMR fails to detect this atom.

*Carbon 13*: The carbon 13 nuclide has one extra (unpaired) neutron and a magnetic field is present in the same way as a single (unpaired) proton produces a field around the hydrogen nucleus.

### Protons in a magnetic field

To produce an NMR signal from protons (or any other paramagnetic nuclei) they must first be exposed to a strong external magnetic field in which they behave like small spinning magnets. In fact, only a small proportion of protons are able to align with the external field because a number of other factors also affect the proton spins. This explains why the NMR signal, even from protons, is comparatively weak and requires the use of very sensitive receivers for its detection.

A freely suspended bar magnet or a magnetized compass needle orientates with its axis parallel to an applied magnetic field. This is due to an interaction between the applied field and the field surrounding the magnetized object. Similarly, a proton will also attempt to align its magnetic axis parallel to an external field. The proton spin creates an additional force which causes its axis to describe a circle around the direction in which it is pointing. This action is termed precession. A practical example can be observed as a spinning top slowly comes to rest in the earth's gravitational field.

### Characteristic frequency

The number of times a nucleus precesses in one second is called the precessional frequency (or Larmor frequency). This is an important distinguishing characteristic of a nucleus. For instance, in a magnetic field of given strength, all the hydrogen nuclei (single protons) will precess at the same frequency. Other types of nuclei will precess at their own characteristic frequencies, which will differ from that of hydrogen nuclei and each other.

Another major factor in determining the value of precessional frequencies is the strength of the applied field. Magnetic field strength is measured in tesla (the SI unit of magnetic flux density) and fields used for MRI generally range from 0.02 to 2.0 tesla. These are very strong compared to the earth's dipole field which is approximately $5 \times 10^{-5}$ tesla. Precessional frequency increases as the magnetic field becomes stronger and is significant in the production of an NMR signal. Table 17.1 gives some examples of magnetic field strength and resultant precessional frequencies for protons (hydrogen nuclei) carbon 13, and phosphorus 31. It can be seen that precessional frequency increases as the magnetic field becomes stronger. There is a basic equation which relates these factors and is given at the end of the chapter, for those who are interested.

## 17.3 The NMR signal

The source of the NMR signal is a weak magnetization through the body, as protons spin (and precess) under the influence of an external magnetic field. As the protons are now pointing in the same general direction, the individual magnetic fields add to each other to produce this extra magnetization.

**Table 17.1** The approximate precessional frequencies of protons, carbon 13 and phosphorus 31, at different magnetic field strengths.

| Magnetic field strength (tesla) | Precessional frequency in MHz | | |
|---|---|---|---|
| | $^1H$ | $^{13}C$ | $^{31}p$ |
| 0.5 | 21.2 | 5.3 | 8.6 |
| 1.0 | 42.6 | 10.7 | 17.2 |
| 1.5 | 63.8 | 16.0 | 25.8 |
| 2.0 | 85.2 | 21.4 | 34.4 |

This represents the total magnetic effect produced by protons spinning in a magnetic field. This magnetization is a vector.

Where the magnetization vector is in the same direction as the applied field, magnetic equilibrium exists. In this situation, the magnetization is undetectable and must be made to change in some way if it is to be recorded.

## Generating the NMR signal

When protons are in magnetic equilibrium, they are spinning in the lowest of two possible energy states. Protons can be excited to a higher energy state where they spin with their axes pointing in the opposite direction. This causes an alteration to their total magnetic effect and a detectable change in the direction of the magnetization vector.

The NMR signal information is recorded following excitation and subsequent deflection of the magnetization vector.

## Excitation and resonance

Excitation can only happen when the protons are able to absorb the precise value of energy for their transition to the higher energy state. In NMR, resonance is where the frequency of the incoming energy exactly matches the frequency of the precessions. Under these conditions, excitation occurs. In practice, this is achieved by exposing the protons to electromagnetic radiation of radio frequency (RF) in order to match the range of proton precessional frequencies.

## Detecting the signal

The exposure to radio waves can swing the magnetization vector through any angle, but useful measurements are made following either a 90° or a 180° deflection. Fig. 17.3(b) shows a 90° deflection caused by a precise radio frequency exposure called the 90° RF pulse. The magnetization vector rotates as the protons spin. This induces a signal voltage in nearby detector

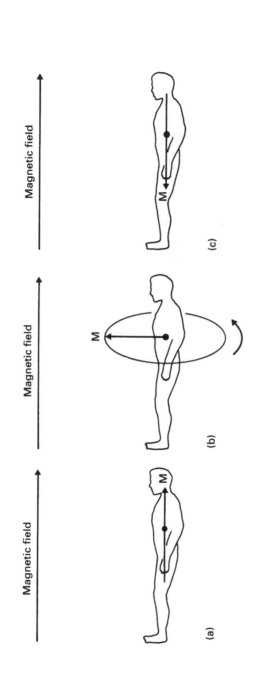

**Fig. 17.3** The direction of nuclear magnetization. The source of the NMR signal is a weak magnetization through the body as protons spin (and precess) under the influence of a magnetic field. As the protons are now pointing in the same general direction, the individual magnetic fields add to each other to produce this extra magnetization. This represents the total magnetic effect produced by protons spinning in a magnetic field. This magnetization is a vector and is represented by the arrow M. (a) In equilibrium. Where the magnetization vector is in the same direction as the applied field, there is a state of magnetic equilibrium. In this situation, the magnetization is undetectable. It must therefore be made to change in some way if it is to be recorded. This is achieved by excitation and subsequent deflection of the magnetization vector. Exposure to radio waves can swing the magnetization vector through any angle, but useful measurements are made following either a 90° or a 180° deflection. (b) Rotating at 90° to the magnetic field, after the 90° radio frequency (RF) pulse. The magnetization vector, shown rotating as the protons spin, induces a signal voltage in nearby detector coils so that information can be collected. Because it is rotating at the same frequency as the protons' precession, the magnetization vector is termed the RF signal. (c) At 180° to the magnetic field, after the 180° RF pulse. When the longer, 180° RF pulse terminates, all protons have been excited and the resultant magnetization is in the opposite direction to the applied field. The signal cannot be detected whilst magnetization is at 180°, but important information is obtained subsequently.

coils so that information can be collected. Because the magnetization vector is rotating at the same frequency as the protons are precessing, it is termed the RF signal.

Fig. 17.3(c) shows the magnetisation vector after the longer 180° RF pulse. When the RF pulse terminates, all protons have been excited and the resultant magnetization is in the opposite direction to the applied field. The signal cannot be detected whilst magnetization is at 180°, but important information is obtained subsequently.

The 90° and 180° RF pulses will initiate different types of signal. Once a signal is detected, the time taken for it to fade away is measured. This process does not happen instantly and is called relaxation. Relaxation times provide key information about the biochemical environment for MR image formation.

### Relaxation times

The physical and chemical factors which determine relaxation times are different for each of these two measurements. After the RF pulse, relaxation is complete when the protons have returned to the lower energy state (and magnetization is back to equilibrium). This process will depend on how quickly the protons can transfer their excess energy to the surroundings. The time measurement is termed relaxation time $T_1$ and gives information about the physical state of the subject.

The RF pulse also gives rise to relaxation where the interaction of adjacent nuclear spins is the major influence on the relaxation time. The signal dies away as the magnetic fields of different atoms interfere with each other and this measurement is termed relaxation time $T_2$. $T_2$ conveys information about the nature of the biochemical surroundings.

## 17.4 The MR image

The MR image is constructed from NMR signals of free hydrogen. However, hydrogen is fairly evenly distributed throughout the body and contrast between tissues is not simply due to changes in hydrogen density. The dramatic contrast, associated with MR images, results because relaxation times are not the same for different types of tissue. Changes in relaxation time are also detected between normal and diseased tissues.

Computer programmed pulse sequences control the imaging process. A sequence employs various combinations of 180° and 90° RF pulses to construct images biased towards either $T_1$ or $T_2$ relaxation characteristics.

Cortical bone cannot be directly imaged by MRI because the hydrogen is too tightly bound. Computed tomography and radiography complement MRI, to evaluate bone lesions. However, bone is surrounded by soft tissue and filled with fatty marrow which does give a strong signal. Active bone

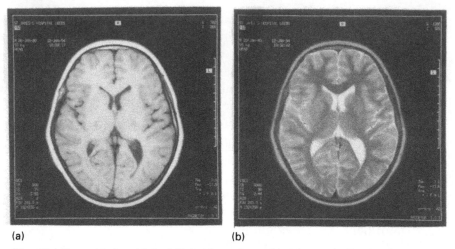

(a)                                          (b)

**Fig. 17.4** Image biasing. (a) An MR head scan image biased towards $T_1$ relaxation characteristics. (b) An MR head scan image biased towards $T_2$ relaxation characteristics. (Contrast can be further enhanced by variations within a particular pulse sequence.) (*Reproduced courtesy of St James's University Hospital, Leeds.*)

lesions will also have cellular matter which will yield a signal. Therefore, the general structure of bone can be visualized as a silhouette against the surrounding tissue signal.

## 17.5  MR scanners

A typical MR scanner has dual couch controls, either side of the central patient tube which passes into the magnet. Three halogen positioning lights are mounted at the opening of the patient tube (located at 9 o'clock, 12 o'clock and 3 o'clock). The patient is moved on the sliding couch top into the magnet for scanning. The couch is of non-ferrous construction to prevent interference with the magnetic field; the top is commonly made of plastic, reinforced with fibreglass.

The design technology of MR scanners advances continually. The object of this section is to explain the essential components of an imaging system at a general practical level.

### The magnet

The magnet produces the strong magnetic field needed for MRI. A magnet is designed to operate at a particular field strength and would fall into one of the following general classifications:

- Low field: less than 0.3 tesla
- Medium field: 0.3 to 1.0 tesla
- High field: greater than 1.0 tesla

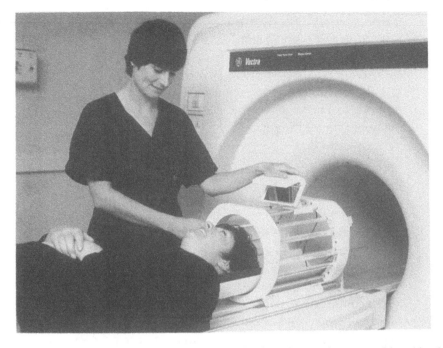

**Fig. 17.5** A typical magnetic resonance scanner. Dual couch controls are seen either side of the central patient tube which passes into the magnet. Three halogen positioning lights are mounted at the opening of the patient tube (located at 9 o'clock, 12 o'clock and 3 o'clock). (*By courtesy of IGE Medical Systems and Lister Bestcare.*)

The choice of magnet strength is not straightforward because there is no simple relationship between field strength and image quality. The advantages of high field techniques can be balanced against costly technical problems in containing a strong magnetic field. It should be noted that high quality images can also be obtained from low and medium field units.

As a result, high, medium and low field systems are in use. Some systems are available which can operate at one strength for imaging (e.g. 1.0 tesla) and at a higher level for spectroscopy (e.g. 2.0 tesla). This alteration takes some time and so field strength would only be changed occasionally.

### Types of magnet

Three types of magnet may be used for MRI:

- Resistive;
- Permanent;
- Superconducting.

### Resistive magnets

The resistive magnet has four or six coils made from aluminium strips.

When an electrical current is passed through the coils, they behave like a large, air-cored solenoid and a magnetic field is generated. (These magnets receive their name from the electrical resistance offered whilst the coils are energized.)

Although the magnet is water cooled, it is difficult to stabilize the current, resulting in fluctuations of the field. These magnets operate up to a maximum of about 0.15 tesla.

### Permanent magnets

A permanent magnet is a large iron horseshoe magnet. These magnets are less expensive to operate and give a low field strength which is stable. They also tend to have a wider central bore. This type of magnet may be found in use – and they produce reasonable quality images. The main problem is that they can weigh up to 20 tons. The installation site must therefore have suitable weight bearing capacity.

### Superconducting magnets

Most modern magnets are of the superconducting type (*supercons*) and have some important advantages. Supercons are able to produce a very stable and uniform magnetic field which is essential for high quality imaging. They can also be manufactured for low, medium or high field techniques.

These magnets employ superconductivity to sustain the magnetic field. This requires the coils to be kept at a very low temperature in a special unit called a cryostat.

### *Superconductivity and cryostats*

Superconductivity is a special property of certain materials. When such a material is cooled to a very low temperature its electrical resistance becomes zero and large currents can flow virtually unimpaired.

When the magnet has been supercooled, a power supply is connected to induce a current in the coils. Electrons flowing in the coil are now in an energy state such that, when the power supply is removed, the current continues to flow. This current and its associated magnetic field remain stable as long as the coils stay cold. Therefore, even when the electrical supply to the scanner is switched off, there is still a field surrounding a superconducting magnet.

The coils of a superconducting magnet are made from fine strands of a niobium and titanium alloy which has superconducting properties at low temperatures. The coils are surrounded by a cooling system called a cryostat. The shields protecting the coils from external heat are made from materials of low thermal conductivity such as stainless steel or fibreglass. The dimensions of the cavities restrict convection and the surfaces are

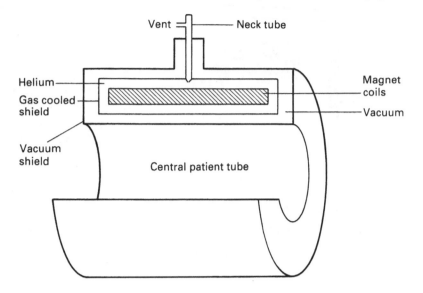

**Fig. 17.6** Section through a supercon cryostat which is cooled by helium. The coils are immersed in liquid helium which carries heat away as it evaporates, at a temperature of 4 K. The helium gas circulates around the gas cooled shield and escapes via the neck tube to a vent above the unit. The surrounding vacuum shield transmits only small amounts of thermal radiation arising from its contact with the atmosphere. The shields protecting the coils from external heat are made from materials of low thermal conductivity such as stainless steel or fibreglass. The dimensions of the cavities restrict convection and surfaces are highly polished to limit heating by radiation transfer.

highly polished to limit heating by radiation transfer (the major source of external heating).

The coils are cooled by immersion in liquid helium. Heat is carried away as the helium evaporates at a temperature of 4 K. The helium gas circulates around the gas cooled shield and escapes via the neck tube, to a vent above the unit. The helium boils off at less than 0.075 litres per hour, but must be replenished at regular intervals of about 12 to 14 weeks.

In older units, helium loss is reduced by a second shield cooled with liquid nitrogen which evaporates at a temperature of 77 K. Developments in refrigerating and recycling systems limit liquid gas losses and modern magnets do not require the nitrogen coolant. Finally there is an outer vacuum shield which protects the inner components. It transmits only small amounts of thermal radiation arising from its contact with the atmosphere.

The following components which lie inside the bore of the main magnet are also electromagnetic coils.

### Shimming

Once the magnet is in operation, the useful field passes through the central

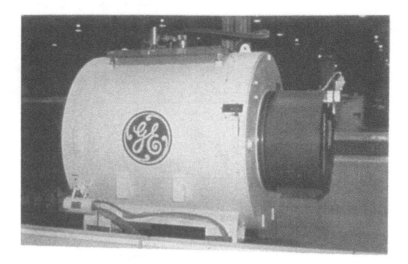

**Fig. 17.7 A superconducting magnet and electrical** coils. The assembly protruding from the main magnet contains electrical coils which control the imaging process. This assembly is fully inside the magnet when installed. (*By courtesy of IGE Medical Systems.*)

bore where the patient tube is located. The field also extends into the surrounding space where it is termed the *fringe field*. The supporting steel structure (yoke) of the magnet, and other steel structures within the room, also become magnetized. This could interfere with the useful field, causing it to become non-uniform.

Compensation for this interference is achieved by **shimming**. One method of shimming is to place a set of shim coils within the bore of the main magnet. The current flowing in these coils is finely controlled to maintain the uniformity of the useful field. Shim coils may also be super-conducting and located in the cryostat.

Shimming may also be achieved through careful design of the supporting framework (passive shimming).

### Magnetic field gradients and gradient coils

A magnetic field gradient exists where the field becomes progressively stronger in a particular direction. The direction of a field strength gradient should not be confused with the direction (polarity) of the field itself. In practice, a magnetic field gradient is produced by imposing a weaker field upon the main field in a controlled way. The weaker field is generated by the gradient coils and either adds to or subtracts from the main field. During the imaging process, gradients are applied in three basic directions which are

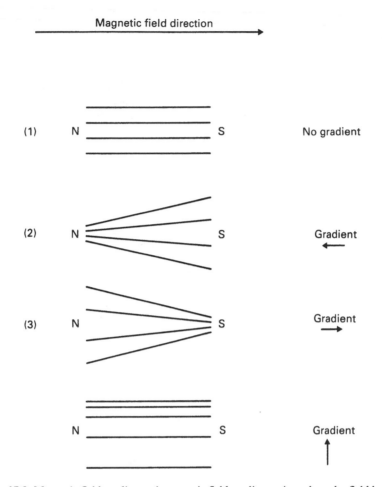

Magnetic field direction

(1)    N ——————— S    No gradient

(2)    N ——————— S    Gradient
                                           ←

(3)    N ——————— S    Gradient
                                           →

        N ——————— S    Gradient
                                           ↑

**Fig. 17.8** Magnetic field gradients. A magnetic field gradient exists where the field becomes progressively stronger in a particular direction. The direction of a field strength gradient should not be confused with the direction (polarity) of the field itself. The simple flux lines represent various gradients imposed on a field. Where the lines are closer the field is stronger.

given the co-ordinates $x$, $y$ and $z$. These gradients localize the image plane and encode the signal for image reconstruction.

Gradients produce a progressive increase in the precessional frequency of protons in given directions. RF pulses are only resonant within a narrow volume of tissue and signals are only received from this thin section. The image slice is selected in this way. Imaging other slices is usually achieved by altering the RF, which is then resonant at different distances along a gradient. There is another, more complex function which may be summarized by saying that after the RF pulse and slice selection, the remaining gradients encode the signal for image reconstruction.

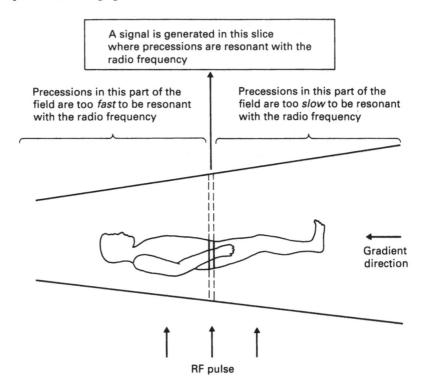

**Fig. 17.9** Localization of a transverse axial plane. A transverse axial plane is shown, localized by a gradient along the length of the body. The gradient produces a progressive increase in the precessional frequency of protons in a certain direction. The RF pulse will only be resonant within a narrow volume of tissue and signals are only received from this thin section. The image slice is selected in this way. Imaging other slices is usually achieved by altering the radio frequency, which is then resonant at different distances along the gradient.

Table 17.2 gives the orientation of the three gradients and Table 17.3 shows the typical functions. Sagittal, axial, coronal and oblique sections can all be imaged without disturbing the patient or requiring any moving mechanical parts. This is a major advantage of MRI. The three gradient coils are located around the patient tube. They may be water or air cooled to prevent overheating.

**Table 17.2** Orientation of magnetic field gradients in imaging.

| Gradient | Typical direction |
|:---:|:---:|
| z | Longitudinal |
| y | Vertical |
| x | Horizontal |

**Table 17.3** Functions of magnetic field gradients in imaging for a horizontal magnetic field.

| Section images | Section selected by | Encoding gradients |
|---|:---:|:---:|
| Axial | z | xy |
| Sagittal | x | yz |
| Coronal | y | xz |
| Oblique | Combinations | Combinations |

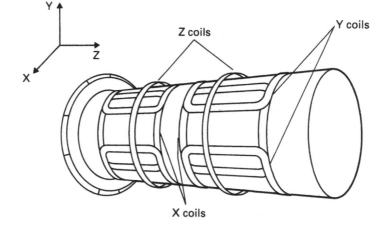

**Fig. 17.10** Gradient coils. The three gradient coils are located as shown, around the patient tube, within the central bore of the main magnet. They may be water cooled or air cooled, to prevent overheating.

## The RF transmitter coils

The coils which emit the RF pulse are situated inside the gradient coils. The RF pulse must be precisely synthesized because it serves a number of important functions:

- Excitation of protons to produce the MR signal.
- The duration of its transmission will determine the flip angle (e.g. a 90° or 180° RF pulse).
- The level of the image slice is determined by the mean frequency of the RF pulse, in association with the slice selecting gradient.
- The thickness of the visualized section is determined by the number of extra frequency components included in the pulse. The section will become thicker as more frequencies are contained in the RF pulse.

Digital RF generators are preferred as they offer the finest control over the critical RF parameters of signal amplitude, frequency and phase.

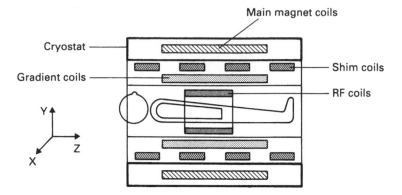

**Fig. 17.11** Diagrammatic section to show relative positions of the main control coils in an MR scanner.

Powering the gradient and RF coils gives rise to a banging sound during operation. This noise is louder in stronger magnets and can be irritating for patients.

## The signal receiver coils

It is important to position the receiver coils as close to the patient as possible in order to detect the signal at its strongest. For this reason a number of different receivers are available. The largest, detecting signals from the body, may be mounted on the same assembly as the RF coils. There will also be a smaller set of head coils and a variety of surface coils. Surface coils are designed to fit directly to the patient's skin and are responsible for the high resolution images now produced.

Some coils transmit the RF signal, as well as receiving it. Modern head coils and extremity surface coils are examples of the transmit/receive type.

## Shielding

Three types of protective shielding must be considered:

- Room RF shielding: protecting the signal receiver coils from interference.
- Magnetic field shielding: protecting surrounding areas from the magnetic field.
- Gradient coil shielding: protecting the imaging field from the effects of induced eddy currents.

### Room RF shielding

Despite the use of surface coils, the best MR signal is still relatively weak

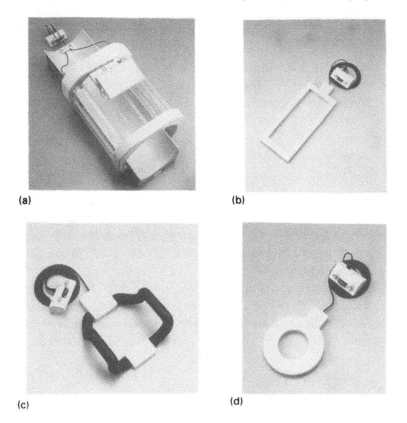

**Fig. 17.12** Signal coils designed to fit directly on the patient's skin. (a) A set of head coils. Head coils can also be seen fitted to the scanner in Fig. 17.5. (b) A transmit/receive wrist coil. (c) A rectangular surface coil (spinal imaging). (d) A coil shaped to fit around the neck. Receiver coils must be as close to the patient as possible, in order to detect the signal at its strongest. The largest, detecting signals from the body, may be mounted on the same assembly as the RF coils. Additionally, however, there are smaller head coils and surface coils, some of which transmit the RF signal, as well as receiving it. These are designed to fit directly to the patient's skin and are responsible for the high resolution images now produced. (*By courtesy of IGE Medical Systems.*)

against background radio noise occurring at similar frequencies. The signal to noise (S/N) ratio is a factor which commands much attention in the design of MR hardware and software. The object is to obtain the best signal with minimum interference.

The scanner is protected by special metal screening built into the walls, floor and ceiling of the scanner room. Openings for doors, vents, electrical supplies and other services such as piped gases must be designed so that they do not disturb the RF shielding.

## Magnetic field shielding
The magnetic field surrounding the magnet can be reduced to safe levels by

shielding and distance. Magnetic field shielding can be of two types: passive and active.

- Passive: the outside of the magnet is clad with steel sheets which are 15 to 20 cm thick. This absorbs the magnetic field directed outwards, but makes the magnet very heavy.
- Active: an additional set of supercooled coils is installed around the main magnet coils, in the cryostat. The field from these coils inhibits the magnetic field directed outwards.

### Gradient coil shielding

The current flowing in the gradient coils is changing rapidly to produce the field gradient pulses during imaging. This induces eddy currents in the surrounding metal structures and these can cause magnetic fields which disturb the main field.

One method of dealing with this is to have matched pairs of gradient coils. The inner (primary) coil produces the gradient imaging pulses. The outer (secondary) coil opposes magnetic flux which would otherwise generate the problem eddy currents. This gradient coil shielding prevents eddy currents occurring.

## 17.6  Control of the imaging process

A computer is essential for controlling the sequence of magnetic field gradients, RF pulses and the acquisition of data for image reconstruction. MR imaging owes its tremendous versatility to the variety of programming software now available.

The program controlling the imaging process governs what is called the *pulse sequence*. The simplest of these is the free induction decay (FID) sequence. This commences with a 90° RF pulse whilst the first slice selecting gradient is applied. The signal is subject to the effects of proton density and is encoded by further gradients for image reconstruction. There follows a recovery period which allows protons in an excited state to settle in equilibrium before the next sequence. This period is also known as the *recovery time (TR)*.

The entire sequence occurs in less than 150 milliseconds, but one FID is not enough for image formation. To collect sufficient data for an image, a minimum of one sequence to every picture element (pixel) is required. A picture matrix of 256 × 256 pixels needs 65 536 ($256^2$) repetitions of the sequence.

To improve the quality of the image the entire set of sequences may be

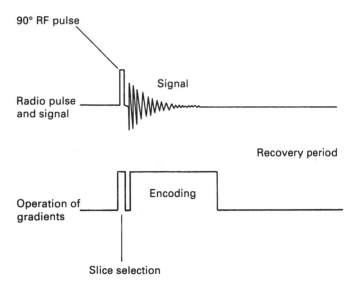

**Fig. 17.13** The free induction decay (FID) pulse sequence. The program controlling the imaging process governs what is called the pulse sequence. The simplest of these is the free induction decay (FID) sequence. This commences with a 90° RF pulse whilst the first slice selecting gradient is applied. The signal is subject to the effects of proton density and is encoded by further gradients for image reconstruction. There follows a recovery period which allows protons in an excited state, to settle in equilibrium before the next sequence. This period is also known as the recovery time (TR).

repeated two to four times and averages of the collected data result in lower noise levels. This is very time consuming.

When selecting techniques, a compromise must be made between the large number of complex sequences needed for high quality images and the long scanning times this would require. Many sequences and operations are being created to reduce scanning time whilst retaining high image quality and it is now possible to produce a series of eight good images in under three minutes.

There are many pulse sequences with a variety of names. The following list gives a brief introduction to some long standing sequences on which many of the newer versions are based.

(1) Free induction decay (FID). This simple sequence does not compensate for interactions between spinning protons. As a result, FID cannot accurately record $T_2$ relaxation. The slightly shorter relaxation it records is referred to as $T_2{}^*$.

(2) Spin echo (SE). This sequence accurately records $T_2$ or $T_1$ relaxation. Recording of $T_1$ or $T_2$ depends on the settings for recovery time (TR) and another period in the sequence called the echo time (TE).

(3) Inversion recovery (IR). This sequence records images based on $T_1$ relaxation times.

There are a number of *fast gradient echo* sequences. They are used for rapid data collection but go by a variety of generic names. This variety in names is because manufacturers adopt their own titles for sequences available on their units.

### Gating

Artefacts may occur when examining organs which contain flowing blood or cerebrospinal fluid. Gating is employed to overcome these artefacts when imaging structures such as the heart and spine.

The scanner is connected, through ECG leads, to a cardiac monitor. This triggers the sequence at the same point in every cardiac cycle to obtain a *still* image. For instance, a rapid imaging sequence is initiated at each R-wave on the ECG.

Respiratory compensation and gating can be used to eliminate artefacts arising from breathing movements. Peripheral gating is where a sensor, known as a photo-plethysmograph, is fitted around the patient's finger or toe. This accessory is easily fitted and provides a gating signal to synchronize data collection by detecting the peripheral circulation. It is used to eliminate artefacts arising from the pulsatile flow of blood or CSF when imaging central nervous system structures. This method of gating is not well suited for cardiac imaging because capillary perfusion in the peripheral tissues affects the timing of the gating signal.

## 17.7 The MR system

When an imaging pulse sequence is initiated, the computer program will trigger the radio pulse synthesizer and gradient amplifiers accordingly. In turn these will energize the RF and gradient coils which generates a signal from the patient. The signals are detected by the receiver coil and pass through the preamplifier on the way to the computer. The signals are digitized and stored in the RAM until enough data has been collected to run the reconstruction program. The image can now be viewed or manipulated at the console and hard copy made.

Permanent storage onto magnetic or optical disk is also possible, but these units must lie outside the influence of the fringe field.

### *The installation*

A room must be chosen which is large enough, receives the necessary services and is capable of bearing the weight of the magnet. Magnets are

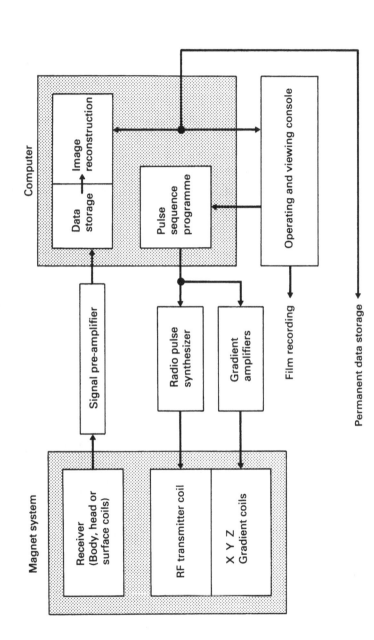

**Fig. 17.14** Basic overview of an MRI system. When an imaging pulse sequence is initiated, the computer program triggers the radio pulse synthesizer and gradient amplifiers accordingly. In turn, these energize the RF and gradient coils which generate a signal from the patient. The signals are detected by the receiver coil and pass through the preamplifier on the way to the computer. The signals are then digitized and stored in the computer's RAM until enough data has been collected to run the reconstruction program. The image can now be viewed or manipulated at the console and hard copy made. Permanent storage onto magnetic or optical disk is also possible, but these units must lie outside the influence of the fringe field.

sited away from roads or lifts as large moving steel masses can disturb the field.

Considerable care must also be taken with regard to any fringe field. Magnets are not usually sited too close to equipment using slow electron beams. Examples of such equipment are electron microscopes, image intensifiers or gamma cameras (photomultiplier tubes are sensitive).

Public areas are protected so that any field is below $5 \times 10^{-4}$ tesla (sometimes called the 5 gauss limit). This is significant as fields above this level are known to interfere with cardiac pacemakers. Clear warning signals are displayed at the entrance to MR suites and security measures are taken to ensure that an unauthorized person could not wander into the magnet room.

The fringe field is three-dimensional and so areas above and below must be considered as well as to the side. The dimensions of the examination room into which an MR unit is installed must be such that the 5 gauss limit, for a fully shielded magnet, lies within the room. The control console must be situated so that the patient can be seen through the observation window.

### Oxygen monitoring

There is usually a monitor set high up in the magnet room which would sound an alarm if the oxygen content fell below about 12%. This is in case of

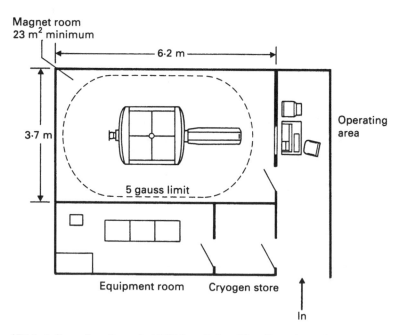

Fig. 17.15 A floor plan of a typical MR installation. The dimensions of the examination room are such that the 5 gauss limit, for a fully shielded magnet, lies within the room. The control console is situated so that the patient can be seen through the observation window.

a large leak of cryogenic gas into the room. As the room fills with gas, oxygen will be displaced downwards and the alarm will be triggered. Cryogenic gas could cause suffocation due to lack of oxygen and is extremely cold.

The cryogen gas may be released on purpose, when *quenching* the magnet. This terminates the magnetic field if necessary and the venting system is designed to cope with the event. Accidental quenching may occur if the temperature within the cryostat is increased for some reason. Accidental quenching is extremely rare.

### Observing the patient

The patient may be observed by a TV camera directed along the bore of the magnet and by setting the control console where a good view of the patient is obtained. Communication with the patient is maintained through a two-way microphone and speaker system.

It can be a claustrophobic experience for the patient and many systems also have a call button for the patient's sense of security. Because there is no hazard from ionizing radiation, friends or relatives who have been screened for pacemakers and loose metal objects (see the section on safety considerations, below) may accompany the patient.

### Changing room requirement

There should be a secure patient changing room outside the influence of the magnetic field because some credit cards may be damaged by magnetism. The patient must remove all metal objects and change into a gown because even a small steel clip could distort the image.

### Quality assurance

Quality assurance is essential to ensure that image construction and relaxation time measurements remain accurate. Special phantoms are of plastic and contain fluids with paramagnetic impurities such as copper sulphate. These are used regularly to assess the imaging process.

## 17.8 Safety considerations

Although there are no hazards from ionizing radiation, there are hazards arising from the use of strong magnetic fields. Careful screening is required for staff, patients and others who will enter the magnet room. The National Radiological Protection Board (NRPB) has laid down detailed safety regulations which govern the exposure to magnetic and radio fields for patients and staff.

The following is a summary of the main regulations and the reasons for each.

## General safety

(1) Access by patients and the public must be restricted.

(2) No small, loose metal objects are allowed into the magnet room. The strength of the magnetic field must not be underestimated. Scissors, needles, screwdrivers and other metal objects have been pulled off trolleys or out of pockets. They are drawn through the air at considerable velocity and can cause serious injury to anyone in the way, or damage to the magnet on impact. This is the missile effect. Metal detectors may be placed at the doors as a precaution against entry with metal objects or trolleys.

(3) There must be special counselling and systems of work for all staff. With the majority of systems, the magnetic field is permanently present. All clinical, domestic, maintenance and emergency procedures (i.e. fire or cardiac arrest) must be well planned to avoid hazards created by the missile effect or entry of personnel who have cardiac pacemakers.

## Some restrictions on techniques

(4) MRI is avoided during the first three months of pregnancy. No adverse effects have been recorded on a fetus, but the same caution is used that applies to the exposure of the fetus to ionizing radiation.

(5) MRI is contraindicated for patients with cardiac pacemakers.

(6) MRI is contraindicated for patients with paramagnetic surgical clips.

(7) Patients with a metal prosthesis should be observed and the examination halted if discomfort is caused.

(8) Resuscitation equipment must be available.

Exposure to strong magnetic fields is now known to cause short term memory loss. Further regulations, which restrict exposure to magnetic and radio fields, are likely.

## Restriction of the magnetic field

(9) Maximum field strength for whole body exposure = 2.0 tesla. Field strengths of above 2.5 tesla can depolarize myocardial cells, which can

lead to arhythmias or cardiac arrest. Higher fields (up to about 4.0 tesla) are allowed if localized to small areas of the limbs. These are normally used for spectroscopy.

(10) The rate at which the magnetic field gradients are changed is limited. A changing magnetic field can induce an emf in nerves which creates some very unpleasant stimuli. Nerve interference can cause involuntary spasms, twitching, or strange sensations. Optic nerve stimulation causes visual disturbances.

The rate at which gradients can change is measured in tesla per second. The maximum rate depends on the strength of the field and the type of pulse sequence.

(11) The body temperature must not be raised by more than $1°C$. The absorption of RF energy causes heating. Raising the body temperature could cause serious illness and must be avoided. The maximum whole body temperature rise of $1°C$ equates to an average power absorption of about 0.4 W/kg. The eye lens is sensitive to heating and cataracts can be caused. The maximum localized power absorption for the eye lens is 100 W/kg (0.1 W/g).

## Protection of staff

(12) Occupational exposure to RF fields should not cause a body temperature rise greater than $1°C$. The operating console is shielded and the area monitored to ensure that the power of any field to which operators may be exposed is below 0.4 W/kg. This equates to a free space incident intensity of 1 mW/cm$^2$.

## 17.9 The NMR equation

$$f_L = \frac{\gamma H_o}{2\pi}$$

where

    $f_L$ = precessional frequency
    $H_o$ = magnetic field strength
    $\gamma$ = gyromagnetic ratio: a constant which relates the physical properties of a particular nucleus to the magnetic field strength

Take the gyromagnetic ratio for protons to be 267.5 which gives the resonant frequency in MHz.

## 17.10 Follow-up practical

As with radionuclide imaging and ultrasound imaging, student radiographers must see, first-hand, the technology and the whole service. Again, the comment is offered that comparisons and contrasts with diagnostic radiography may prove valuable.

# Index

CPSIA information can be obtained
at www.ICGtesting.com
Printed in the USA
FSHW020154031220
76349FS